# All in Your Head

The publisher gratefully acknowledges the generous support of the General Endowment Fund of the University of California Press Foundation.

# All in Your Head

Making Sense of Pediatric Pain

## Mara Buchbinder

UNIVERSITY OF CALIFORNIA PRESS

University of California Press, one of the most distinguished university presses in the United States, enriches
lives around the world by advancing scholarship in the
humanities, social sciences, and natural sciences. Its
activities are supported by the UC Press Foundation and
by philanthropic contributions from individuals and
institutions. For more information, visit www.ucpress.edu.

University of California Press
Oakland, California

Library of Congress Cataloging-in-Publication Data

Buchbinder, Mara, author.
   All in your head : making sense of pediatric pain /
Mara Buchbinder.
      pages   cm.
   Includes bibliographical references and index.
   ISBN 978–0-520–28521–7 (cloth : alk. paper)
   ISBN 978–0-520–28522–4 (pbk. : alk. paper)
   ISBN 978–0-520–96076–3 (ebook)
   1. Pain in children.   2. Pain in children—Social
aspects.   3. Pain—Social aspects.   4. Pain clinics—
United States.   I. Title.
   RJ365.B83   2015
   618.92'0472—dc23

                                          2014044788

Manufactured in the United States of America

24   23   22   21   20   19   18   17   16   15
10   9   8   7   6   5   4   3   2   1

*for Simon Joseph*

# Contents

# Acknowledgments

This book considers what can be gained by thinking about chronic pain not only as a private experience, but also as one that is managed, explained, and understood in deeply relational ways. Much like chronic pain, I have found writing a book to be a much more social endeavor than is often assumed. Insights, introductions, kindnesses, and conversations offered by my colleagues, mentors, family, and friends have left a profound impression on me and on my research, and have helped to shape the story I have to tell in the pages that follow.

My greatest debt is to the clinicians, patients, and families who welcomed me into their worlds and shared their experience with me. Marcia Meldrum and Ignasi Clemente facilitated the introductions that made this research possible, and I am appreciative of them for supporting this work from the beginning. Although I cannot thank her by name, I am particularly grateful to the person I call "Dr. Novak" for seeing the value of anthropological research on clinical problems and supporting my research from the beginning. I am immensely grateful, too, for the adolescents and families who trusted me during some of their most vulnerable moments and gave so generously to this project.

This book began as a doctoral dissertation, and I could find no better intellectual role models for the specific areas of inquiry that I bring together in this book than the members of my PhD committee at UCLA. Linda Garro and Jason Throop are among the most prominent scholars in the anthropology of pain and have provided gracious, consistent guidance in this area, while Elinor Ochs and John Heritage taught me how to approach language as a fundamental dimension of social life. As dissertation co-chairs, Linda and Ellie offered complementary strengths and made me especially grateful for fortuitously finding an intellectual home during my doctoral training that recognized the productive synergy between medical/psychological and linguistic anthropology. I am especially grateful to Jason for introducing me to Reed Malcolm and helping me to find a home for this book. I also benefited during my graduate training from steady support from a number of other UCLA faculty members, particularly Carole Browner, Stefan Timmermans, Candy Goodwin, and Alessandro Duranti.

I am grateful to the University of North Carolina at Chapel Hill and the broader Triangle area for providing such a warm, generous, and lively intellectual environment for nurturing this book. I could scarcely have imagined landing in such a dynamic spot as a newly minted PhD in medical anthropology. At UNC, I thank my colleagues in the Department of Social Medicine, especially Sue Estroff, Barry Saunders, Raul Necochea, Rebecca Walker, Annie Lyerly, Jill Fisher, Jon Oberlander, Eric Juengst, Arlene Davis, and Department Chair Gail Henderson, and my colleagues in the Department of Anthropology and Moral Economies of Medicine working group, especially Michele Rivkin-Fish, Jocelyn Chua, and Peter Redfield. I also owe a huge debt of gratitude to my local writing partners—Jocelyn Chua, Nadia El-Shaarawi, Lauren Fordyce, Tomas Matza, Saiba Varma, and Harris Solomon—inspiring colleagues and friends who offered valuable criticism as this project was coming to a close. Their camaraderie, support, and generous feedback left me feeling confident and energized about the project during moments of doubt. I am grateful to Nadia for many loops around Duke's East campus and so much more.

My thinking and writing have also benefited tremendously from conversations with and written comments from Steve Black, Paul Brodwin, Beth Bromley, Bambi Chapin, Megan Crawley-Matoka, Hanna Garth, Jennifer Guzman, Mark Luborsky, Cari Merritt, Keith Murphy, Sarah Pinto, Sonya Pritzker, Michele Rivkin-Fish, Rayna Rapp, Sarah Rubin, Andrea Sankar, Merav Shohet, Stefan Timmermans, Kristin Yarris, and Allan Young. Three anonymous reviewers read a complete draft of the book manuscript and offered insightful feedback that pushed me to clarify my arguments and my central intellectual contributions. I am most grateful for their time, efforts, and generous care, which truly represent the pinnacle of unpaid academic labor. I am also grateful to the participants of the 2012 Rise of Child Science and Psy-Expertise workshop at Brunel University and the Royal Anthropological Institute, especially to the organizer, Dominique Behague.

The research on which this book is based was funded by generous support from the National Science Foundation and the Wenner-Gren Foundation for Anthropological Research. Time for writing and thinking was made possible by a scholarly residency at the Brocher Foundation in Hermance, Switzerland, in May 2012, a UNC CTSA Interdisciplinary Clinical Research Career Development Award from the National Institutes of Health (KL2TR001109), and a semester of teaching leave from the Department of Social Medicine at UNC–Chapel Hill. I am also grateful to have received a publication grant from UNC's University Research Council.

I thank Reed Malcolm at the University of California Press for seeing value in this project and for making the editorial process smooth and transparent from start to finish. I am especially grateful to Reed for soliciting such valuable reader reports from my anonymous peer reviewers. Stacey Eisenstark and Rachel Berchten demonstrated the utmost attention and care in guiding the book (and its author) through the production process.

My parents, Harriet and Marty Yogel and Stephen Buchbinder, my sister Emily Hutton, and my in-laws, Catherine and Craig Summers, have been steadfast supporters of my work and gave me space and time to write on many visits home. Among the many members of my extended clan of step-siblings, whom I am very lucky to call family, the chronic pain experiences of my inspiring sister, Diana Falchuk, were never far from my mind when I began working on what became chapter 2 of this book. Diana also played an important role in helping me to launch my research career by introducing me to Michael Rich and Jennifer Patashnick at the Children's Hospital, Boston, where I started the work that became my undergraduate honors thesis. Jesse Summers' discerning eye has scanned every page of this text except for these acknowledgments. I have been lucky to have a partner who continually challenges me to strive for greater clarity, brevity, and humility in my thinking and writing. His greatest gift, however, has been to share his life, and his love, with me.

The dissertation on which this book is based was dedicated to my beloved grandfather, Simeon Joseph Bogin, who passed away weeks after I filed, a few months short of his hundredth birthday. I dedicate this book to his namesake, Simon Joseph Summers, who arrived a few years later and has thus far honored his great-grandfather's memory in every possible way. Thank you, Simon, for filling our home with your boundless curiosity and effervescent laughter, and for giving me a reason to close my laptop and put this project to rest. I hope that you will never know the pain of which these pages tell.

An earlier version of chapter 2 was published as "Personhood Diagnostics: Personal Attributes and Clinical Attributions of Pain," *Medical Anthropology Quarterly* 25, no. 4 (2011). An earlier version of chapter 3 was published as "'Sticky' Brains and Sticky Encounters in a U.S. Pediatric Pain Clinic," *Culture, Medicine, and Psychiatry* 36, no. 1 (2012). Very brief excerpts of the Introduction, chapter 3, and chapter 5 were published in "Neural Imaginaries and Clinical Epistemology: Rhetorically Mapping the Adolescent Brain in the Clinical Encounter," *Social Science and Medicine,* in press (2014). I gratefully acknowledge Wiley-Blackwell, Springer, and Elsevier for providing permission to reprint these materials here in revised form.

# Acronyms and Initialisms

| | |
|---|---|
| ACE | angiotensin-converting enzyme |
| ADD | attention deficit disorder |
| ADHD | attention deficit/hyperactivity disorder |
| ASL | American Sign Language |
| BPD | borderline personality disorder |
| CAM | complementary and alternative medical (therapies) |
| CBT | cognitive behavioral therapy |
| CRPS | chronic regional pain syndrome |
| DSM | *Diagnostic and Statistical Manual of Mental Disorders* |
| EEG | electroencephalogram |
| EKG | electrocardiogram |
| FDA | Food and Drug Administration |
| GATE | Gifted and Talented Education program (California) |
| GI | gastroenterology |
| HMO | health maintenance organization |
| IASP | International Association for the Study of Pain |
| IBS | irritable bowel syndrome |
| IT | information technology |
| MRI | magnetic resonance imaging |

| | |
|---|---|
| OCD | obsessive compulsive disorder |
| PDD | pervasive developmental disorder |
| PDD-NOS | pervasive developmental disorder not otherwise specified |
| RSD | reflex sympathetic dystrophy |
| SSRI | selective serotonin reuptake inhibitor |

# Transcription Conventions

[         indicates overlapping speech

:         indicates phonological elongation

-         indicates a noticeable and abrupt termination of a word or sound

,         indicates a continuing intonation (not necessarily a grammatical comma)

.         indicates a completing intonation (not necessarily a grammatical period)

(.)       indicates a brief pause

=        indicates that one turn runs into another with no interval

(xxx)    indicates indecipherable content

(( ))     indicates nonverbal action

# Introduction

The merest schoolgirl, when she falls in love, has Shakespeare
or Keats to speak her mind for her; but let a sufferer try to
describe a pain in his head to a doctor and language at once
runs dry.

—Virginia Woolf, *On Being Ill*


In what sense are my sensations *private?*—Well, only I can
know whether I am really in pain; another person can only
surmise it.—In one way this is wrong, and in another
nonsense.

—Ludwig Wittgenstein, *Philosophical Investigation*


Marian Grindall wiped a tear from her cheek.[1] "I always feel like I'm
just right on the edge of tears," she said apologetically. Silently, I cursed
myself for again forgetting to bring tissues. I was sitting with Marian
and her husband, Tom, at their kitchen table on a quiet Sunday morning in February. Abundant sunlight streamed in through French doors,
glinting off modern silver appliances and softening their weary faces. I
listened intently as they explained to me how their seventeen-year-old
daughter, Cassandra, their only child, had come down with a mysterious illness in September that had left her bedridden for months with
painful headaches and a dizzying nausea. No one had been able to
diagnose her problem, and the lengthy illness and futile search for an
explanation had taken a toll on the family. Cassandra shut herself in
her bedroom for hours on end, which troubled her parents greatly.
"When she wants something, she knocks on the wall," Marian said.
"It's just a battle to even get her to get up out of bed so I can change her
sheets."

Two months later, a team of clinicians sat around a table in a drab, mauve-painted conference room discussing Cassandra's case. Ted Bridgewater, an acupuncturist, had treated her twice, and was very concerned. Usually, patients relax once the acupuncture needles have been inserted, he said, but Cassandra had remained rigid for the duration of the treatment. Moreover, her tongue was swollen, indicating "stuck dampness," and this was not a good sign.[2] "Part of the problem is that she hasn't bought into us," Ted surmised. Rebecca Hunter, a child and family therapist, was also deeply worried. Her main concern was that Cassandra was convinced that the only way she would get better was if she hid out in her bedroom for three or four weeks. She had cut off all contact with her friends, who served as a reminder that her life was moving on without her. "It's extreme," Rebecca said. "She may end up needing inpatient treatment." Dr. Novak, Cassandra's physician, was alarmed by this suggestion, and resolved to revisit her chart after the meeting so that they could put her case at the top of the list for the next meeting.

Cassandra's case highlights a curious paradox about pain: while it has long been viewed as the quintessential private experience, pain is configured, explained, understood, and even experienced in ways that are deeply relational. Across the humanities and social sciences, scholars have argued that chronic pain is inexpressible, imperceptible, and alienating, and thus essentially unknowable by others. This portrait of pain is poignantly reflected in the image of Cassandra alone in her bedroom, where she remained isolated for weeks on end, cut off from her family and friends. At the same time, however, glimpses of another view of pain emerge in the foregoing scenes. A middle-aged couple tells their daughter's story to a curious anthropologist, and in the telling, convey their own internalization of their daughter's long-term suffering. A group of clinicians meets to discuss a patient's treatment, conveying their care and concern. Without denying that pain is a fundamentally private experience, these two scenes reveal that pain, in some important senses, is also profoundly social.

Phenomenological approaches to pain have flourished in recent years, because pain has been cast as a private experience that shatters language and evades representation.[3] And yet, despite the obvious epistemological constraints on apprehending another's internal states, language is what translates pain from the solitary and unknowable to a phenomenon that is richly and excruciatingly described in literature, medicine, and everyday life. *All in Your Head: Making Sense of Pediat-*

*ric Pain* builds on phenomenological accounts to capture the life-altering dimensions of chronic pain, but situates pain in an intersubjective context to emphasize the relational, everyday means by which it is understood and managed. Through careful attention to the language of pain—including narratives, conversations, models, and metaphors—and detailed analysis of how pain sufferers make meaning through interactions with others, this book reveals that, however private pain may be, making sense of it is deeply social.

In the pages that follow, I draw on ethnographic research that I conducted from 2008 to 2009 in a Southern-California-based multidisciplinary pediatric pain clinic, which I call the West Clinic, to explore how clinicians, adolescent patients, and their families make sense of puzzling symptoms and work to alleviate pain. It is important to state from the outset that this book does not address the embodied experience of pain—what pain *feels* like to those who suffer it—or at least does not do so directly. Several exemplary ethnographies have charted the lived experience of pain in heartrending detail, and I refer interested readers to these works.[4] My primary goal for this book has been somewhat different: to trace the ways in which chronic pain transcends the individual body through its treatment in the social arena. A related goal for this work has been to attend closely to practitioners' discourse and clinical experiences, which are necessarily orthogonal to the phenomenology of pain, and have received relatively less attention than patient perspectives in the social scientific literature.[5]

Where adult chronic pain patients have inspired long-standing debates about whether American society ought to bear the collective burden of lost work and productivity, there are no general expectations in the contemporary United States that children and adolescents make substantial economic contributions to society. Greater, here, is the moral burden of grappling with children's suffering. Middle-class Americans by and large presume that children are innocent, dependent, and vulnerable, and view children's health as an index of societal well-being.[6] While the situation is somewhat more complicated for adolescents, for reasons that I explore in this book, they, too, are presumed to require special safeguards and protections. During my fieldwork, parents constantly told me that they felt horrible about being unable to relieve their children's suffering and wished they could bear their children's pain.

It is precisely this vulnerability that makes pediatric pain a rich case for exploring the social embedding of pain. This book focuses specifically on chronic pain during adolescence, a time of great social upheaval in the United States and elsewhere.[7] For some West Clinic patients, academic pressure, troubles with peers, and strained relations within the family appeared to play an important role in the onset and course of pain. For others, the pain did not seem to be etiologically linked to such stressors, but nevertheless dramatically altered the adolescent's social world and future aspirations once it appeared on the scene. Each of these possibilities strengthens the view that living with chronic pain is a thoroughly social phenomenon, and that managing pain is always deeply rooted in ongoing social life and family care.

To foreground the relational dimensions of pain is to attend to the multiple ways in which empathy seeps through the impenetrability of pain in subtle gestures or carefully selected words. It is also to recognize how caring for people with chronic pain is constituted as an active, engaged, and intimate social practice. Such care comes in many forms. For Marian Grindall, caring for Cassandra meant helping her wash her long, matted hair, after her daughter, who had once taken great pride in her appearance, had all but given up on her hygiene. Marian described how they soaked Cassandra's hair in conditioner and divided it into tiny sections to carefully detangle the mess of knots so that they would not need to cut her hair. It took two painstaking hours to complete the job, but she saved her daughter's hair.

This type of care is all the more crucial for chronic pain patients like Cassandra and other West Clinic patients, who face regular affronts to their sense of self-worth. Because it is invisible, chronic pain is not accountable to the same types of evidentiary truths as the pain of a wound or a broken limb. It therefore renders its subjects morally suspect, calling the authenticity of their suffering into question. Chronic pain thus raises additional challenges to language and belief that people in pain can begin to overcome only when sustaining intimate relationships with others.

The title of this book, *All in Your Head,* references its exploration of two related themes. First, it examines how cultural models of mind and brain are mobilized in explanations of pain.[8] For decades, patients have been told that their pain is "all in your head" when diagnostic tests are negative or inconclusive. Cassandra Grindall had been told this by so many doctors—that there was nothing wrong with her, aside from quite clearly being depressed—that she became completely disillusioned with the field of medicine, and Marian and Tom had to work hard to persuade her to give the West Clinic a chance. However, while explaining pain as "all in your head" sets off instant alarm bells for pain patients, the past few decades have witnessed a dramatic revolution in how pain researchers understand the neurobiology of pain, and the brain now figures centrally in clinical explanations. By analyzing the neuroscientific tropes that clinicians employ in conversation with families, I illustrate that chronic pain is, after all, "in the head"—but not in the way figured by psychosomatic discourse. Instead, the rise of "neuro" explanatory discourses illustrates that all pain can effectively be traced to the brain (in the head), while preserving the patient's legitimacy.

Second, *All in Your Head* addresses long-standing anthropological questions about how people search for meaning and assign blame in the face of adversity. Building on a large body of anthropological work that examines how people make sense of illness and distressing events, I illustrate how different explanatory frameworks for chronic pain are foregrounded by clinicians and families at different points in the therapeutic process. In doing so, I suggest that there is seldom a single explanation for pain, such as "all in your head." Instead, causality is best understood in terms of a shifting constellation of explanatory factors, which are mobilized at different points in the therapeutic process, for different pragmatic purposes.

Marian and Tom located the beginning of Cassandra's troubles in a mysterious, undiagnosed illness that she developed at nine years old, resulting in the rapid loss of more than a third of her body weight. The episode was initially quite worrisome, but Cassandra eventually recovered and regained the weight. A few years later, when the symptoms reemerged, the Grindalls learned that Cassandra had an IgA protein deficiency, a common immune deficiency disorder. For Marian, "that explained to us why she always catches every bug that goes around and just answered a lot of that part of the question for us." When the problems resurfaced again, however, the Grindalls were faced, in Marian's words, with the questions: "Is this related? Is it unrelated? Is it a new problem? Is it an old problem?" They also cited, as possible alternative causes, the toll of her cheerleading competitions, her busy social calendar, and her attempts to earn straight A's at school. Later, many weeks into her treatment, Cassandra's care team raised questions about whether her pain might be caused by an undisclosed trauma. Each of these explanatory factors offers a different interpretive window onto Cassandra's pain, windows we will peer through as we examine the multiple layers of explanation that go into making sense of pain.

## THE PROBLEM OF EXPLANATION

Marian and Tom Grindall were absorbed by the need to explain Cassandra's symptoms because explanation is a fundamental tool for making sense of, and responding to, suffering. Explanations translate disorder into order by assembling events into a causal framework and endowing them with meaning. While explanation is a topic of concern for scholars from a range of disciplines from cognitive science to philosophy, as an anthropologist, I am particularly interested in examining how culture shapes the attribution of meaning and explanatory legitimacy—that is, which explanations are deemed to count—within a specific context. For example, Chinese medicine does not adhere to the same standards of mutual exclusivity and economy of causes that dominate Western scientific causal models.[9] Within anthropology, explanation has been a central focus of what has been referred to as the rationality debates, a set of conversations emerging in the 1960s about how anthropologists should articulate and understand putatively irrational ways of thinking among the people they study, including a critical look at the conceptual language used to ground epistemological claims.[10] This line of inquiry reflects an interlinking set of concerns about the relationship between our ontological assumptions about the world and the social production of knowledge.

Explanation has been a topic of particular interest to medical anthropologists because it plays a crucial role in understanding the culturally grounded ways in which people interpret illness and distress. Along with medicine, magic and religion have held privileged roles as institutional arenas for making sense of misfortune; in fact, the earliest forms of healing emerged in magic and religion. Across a variety of cultural and historical settings, magic has been a valuable resource for explaining the apparently inexplicable, that which eludes conventional scientific frameworks. Early studies of witchcraft and sorcery thus offer useful templates for examining causal reasoning about illness.[11] According to the anthropologist E. E. Evans-Pritchard, for instance, the Zande of north central Africa attribute all misfortunate events to witchcraft unless presented with strong evidence to the contrary. Yet because they recognize a plurality of causes, explanations tied to the natural world do not contradict the mystical causes layered onto such events. In his classic example, Evans-Pritchard suggested that although the Azande know that the collapse of old granaries is caused by the decay of wooden supports eaten by termites, the fact that a *particular* set of people were sitting under such a granary at a *particular* moment in time, sustaining injury during its collapse, is nevertheless attributed to witchcraft. Witchcraft thus explains *why* the granary collapses on someone in addition to *how* it does so.[12]

This book is particularly concerned with the explanatory frameworks employed in contemporary U.S. biomedicine.[13] The notion that medical explanations are culturally constructed hinges on a larger set of claims about medicine itself, and medical language more specifically.[14] In his foundational work, the physician-anthropologist Arthur Kleinman suggested that medicine is first and foremost a cultural system: "a system of symbolic meanings anchored in particular arrangements of social institutions and patterns of interpersonal interactions."[15] By this Kleinman means that medicine is not purely a natural science, but also integrates elements of the human sciences in its social and moral concerns. If medicine is a cultural system like religion or magic, it follows that it can be mined, like any cultural system, for its internal logics, constitutive practices, and repertoires of specialized knowledge.

The language of medicine, likewise, is also culturally shaped. The metaphor of the body as a machine, for example, a key explanatory trope in contemporary biomedicine, reflects a widely shared cultural model of the body as made up of interchangeable—and thus, potentially fixable and/or replaceable—parts.[16] Thus, as the anthropologist Byron Good has put it, "the language of medicine is hardly a simple mirror of the empirical world," but rather is shaped by cultural values and knowledge.[17] The approach to medical language that I adopt in this book suggests that clinical explanations are cultural and historical products that reveal a multitude of coded assumptions about the body and the social world, including ideas about morality, responsibility, and relations between kin.

### Dimensions of Biomedical Explanation

Biomedical explanations encompass at least four significant dimensions.[18] First, biomedical explanations ascribe relations of *cause*. In U.S. biomedicine, the designation of cause is relatively circumscribed, with etiological understandings generally restricted to Aristotle's category of efficient cause: here, the series of events that set a disease in motion.[19] Yet where biomedicine is principally concerned with causes that are located at the individual level, as when a pathogen penetrates the body and produces disease,[20] medical anthropologists have been particularly attentive to causes that originate in the social world. Sherine Hamdy's notion of *political etiologies* underscores the ways in which diseases may be understood as outcomes of social, economic, and political ailments. Hamdy shows how Egyptian patients with kidney failure express political etiologies as part of a set of physical and social grievances.[21] Causal explanations are thus political insofar as they suggest where responsibility and retribution lie. For example, the attribution of symptoms to certain environmental conditions has been the basis for patients' claims of entitlement to compensatory benefits.[22]

Hamdy suggests that a lack of etiological clarity from medical experts makes patients more apt to develop their own causal theories. This brings us to *certainty*, the second key dimension of biomedical explanations. Linguistic devices embedded in biomedical explanations convey a range of epistemic certainty. When a physician says, "Now there appears to be an infection at the contact point of the joint below it in the sac of mucus there in the hip," the evidential verb "appear" expresses the sensory basis for the diagnostic explanation, while signaling that the conclusion is nevertheless somewhat tentative.[23] Similarly, the physician's hedging in the following explanation for chest pain preserves a measure of uncertainty: "Um I think it may be that you know sometimes people get chest pain from other things, from their muscles for example."[24] These statements reveal the interactional production of biomedical uncertainty, while also highlighting how the physician's expertise and authority are managed and performed on the ground.

Third, biomedical explanations relay specific relationships to *truth*. Just as the credibility of certain medical systems, such as Aryurvedic medicine, can be questioned from the standpoint of conventional Western medicine,[25] U.S. biomedicine is not immune to such challenges. An important body of work in science studies has demonstrated that even scientific explanations are not as bound by positivist understandings of truth and evidence as is often assumed.[26] Moreover, the truth of medical explanations may be judged according to different criteria. We may form retrospective judgments about whether explanations accord with what we already think or know, or prospective judgments about whether explanations reflect what is likely to happen in the future.[27] Clinical explanations in U.S. psychiatry often reflect a pragmatic orientation to truth, in which "psychiatrists do not necessarily commit themselves to a particular view on the underlying structure of the universe."[28] Instead, psychiatric explanations are regarded as "true" insofar as they yield positive practical consequences, such as relieving symptoms and promoting therapeutic efficacy.

Finally, biomedical explanations relay how illness happens as well as, to varying degrees, why it occurs. This reveals a concern for *meaning*, the fourth dimension in this typology. While the long-standing focus on patient perspectives within meaning-centered medical anthropology might create the impression that biomedical accounts are impoverished of meaning,[29] anthropological studies reveal a substantial concern with meaning among biomedical practitioners themselves.[30] Meaning is a critical component of biomedical explanations insofar as explanations encode moral judgments about the source of suffering and the patient's deservingness of certain treatments. Ascribing pain to cancer—widely understood to cause tremendous pain and suffering—might suggest that a patient deserves to be given opioid analgesics,[31] while patients with sickle cell disease—a disease that often raises racially charged suspicions of "drug-seeking" and addiction—face extraordinary challenges in obtaining effective treatment.[32] This underscores that explanatory meaning is not only symbolic, but is also embedded in underlying relations of power and structures of inequality.

Threaded through each of the elements is the matter of diagnosis. In the U.S. biomedical context, diagnosis is, in a sense, the ultimate goal of causal reasoning, yet it includes considerations of certainty, truth, and meaning. Consequently, it might make sense to think of diagnosis as the fundamental explanatory act in medicine. However, even this is culturally shaped and not simply given. In Chinese medicine, for example, diagnosis is made after feeling the pulse and is not accompanied by a great deal of explanatory rhetoric.[33] Likewise, in the Yapese bonesetting practices described by the anthropologist Jason Throop, diagnosis is grounded in embodied knowledge and sensorial attunement.[34] In both of these cases, far different from the kind of therapeutic encounters to which we will soon turn, diagnosis is structured by an economy of expression that places more emphasis on tactile engagement than on offering an explanation.

## The Pragmatics of Explanation

Medical explanations consolidate a great deal of social, moral, and medical information. Yet explanations do more than simply represent the world as it is: they are also mobilized for specific social ends. This distinction between language as a tool of reference—that is, the idea that words represent things in the world—and language as a form of social action is embodied in what linguists refer to as the referential and performative functions of language.[35] My own approach to medical explanation hinges on a performative view of language, which emphasizes that language is a pragmatic tool that both reflects and helps to construct sociocultural worlds.

Here, my thinking is influenced by the philosopher of science Evelyn Fox Keller, who has argued for serious attention to the rhetorical dimensions of scientific explanation. Drawing on a close reading of explanatory models and metaphors in the biological sciences, Keller suggests that explanations may best be viewed as "semi-fictions," which work "not so much as a way of guiding us toward a more precise and literal description of phenomena but rather as a way of providing explanatory satisfaction where it is not otherwise available."[36] Following Keller, I suggest that clinical explanations share a close affinity with some forms of scientific models insofar as their utility lies in their heuristic value—that is, the practical meanings that they afford.[37]

Keller also speaks of the multiplicities of epistemological cultures, "the norms and mores of a particular group of scientists that underlie the particular meanings they give to words like theory, knowledge, explanation, and understanding, and even to the concept of practice itself."[38] In this book, I draw on this conceptualization of multiplicity and the pragmatics of meaning, but I also point to the hybridity within (as well as across) particular epistemological cultures. As we will see, patients, their families, and even clinicians themselves do not subscribe to a single, isolatable explanation of pain, but employ different interpretive frameworks for different reasons at different historical moments. In Cassandra Grindall's case, this meant shifting from the investigation of possible viral or immunodeficiency causes to a more difficult exploration, further down the road in her treatment, into whether her symptoms might have traumatic origins.

## EXPLAINING PAIN

Explaining pain, as a particular form of medical explanation, entails particular interpretive and intersubjective challenges deriving from two interrelated problems: pain's status as an inner experience, and the inadequacies of language to capture this experience fully. First, because pain cannot be directly observed, its presence must be inferred through report or behavior. Clinicians read the body for signs that may help them distinguish between patients with real and "unreal" pain—that is, pain that is taken to be nonexistent or made up.[39] Thus, although pain is a private experience, it depends on social action to make it real to others (and hence treatable). To ask about whether one's pain is real is, therefore, an unavoidably social question.

In contemporary biomedicine, vision is a privileged epistemological model for making the body legible. From their earliest experiences in the cadaver lab, neophyte physicians are socialized into new ways of seeing the body, which in turn shape how they see the world.[40] Biomedicine's reliance on this way of knowing is not a natural fact, but rather the product of a specific set of cultural and historical conditions that generated a crucial epistemological shift—from a view in which text-based learning generates medical knowledge to one in which knowledge emanates from the physician's ability to penetrate the body and see its hidden, underlying truths.[41] From this perspective, it is not difficult to see why chronic pain, which all too often evades visual representation through imaging technologies, occupies such a precarious status in biomedicine: in order to know that symptoms are "real," physicians need to be able to see them.

Attempts to decipher whether or not pain is "real" are tied to the tenacious legacy of mind-body dualism in U.S. biomedicine and Western culture more generally. Notions of mind-body dualism build on commonsense, ethnopsychological assumptions about the separation between mental and physical states. Outside of philosophy, much of the scholarly writing on pain presumes that the concept of dualism necessitates that the causes of pain must be either mental or physical, but not both.[42] Western biomedicine has been criticized for perpetuating reductionism and dualism, even though most physicians are not concerned with dualism as a metaphysical problem in their day-to-day practice.[43] Nevertheless, the notion of mind-body dualism in medicine remains a powerful trope in medical anthropology and the medical humanities more broadly, in part because it provides a metaphoric basis for thinking about blame and responsibility for illness. Western culture tends to hold individuals responsible for illnesses of the mind, but less so for illnesses of the body.

Chronic pain is often surrounded by an atmosphere of uncertainty, and even doubt and mistrust. In my earlier work on newborn screening for genetic disorders, Stefan Timmermans and I identified several types of uncertainty at stake in biomedical encounters.[44] Clinicians not only face epistemic uncertainty—about how we can ever really know the source of another person's suffering, and whether she is truly in pain—but also ontological uncertainty about the nature of symptoms and their relationship to diagnostic categories. Families, in particular, but clinicians, too, also face prognostic uncertainty about what illness may mean for a child's future.[45] Each of these types of uncertainty colors the experience of adolescents grappling with chronic pain and their relationships with clinicians and loved ones.

In this book, as in my last, I do not treat uncertainty as a problem to be solved, in detective-like fashion, by applying medical knowledge. This means that I bracket the underlying, often unspoken, issue of whether pain, for any given individual, is "really real."[46] Instead, I suggest that uncertainty is a phenomenon that must be constantly managed in ongoing social interactions: in the clinic, at school, and at home. By focusing on the clinical and social realities of pain management, I explore how clinicians, patients, and families grapple with—and dance around—questions about pain's reality. In doing so, I show how pain is made real by the ways in which we name, frame, and treat it.[47]

At stake for adolescents, in particular, are enduring cultural questions about whether children are to be treated as reliable narrators of their own embodied experience.[48] Adolescents are often viewed with suspicion as clinical actors, and their rationality and judgment are frequently called into question.[49] Are they then seen as possessing the means to determine whether their pain is real? How does their liminal status in American culture influence the evidentiary stature we accord their complaints? Such questions are particularly important in light of the profound social stressors that many American adolescents face, which appear to offer incentives for them to adopt the sick role and avoid their normal activities.

The second key challenge for explaining pain relates to the role of language. While rich vocabularies for describing pain exist in many languages,[50] their ability to convey the experience of pain adequately has been consistently questioned. This resistance to language may relate, in part, to a cultural imperative in many parts of the world to face pain with stoicism.[51] Yet it also concerns the challenges that pain poses for relaying private experience to the outside world. In her foundational text, *The Body in Pain,* the literary critic Elaine Scarry argues that pain resists symbolization through language and is therefore fundamentally inexpressible.[52] According to Scarry, one of the primary reasons for this resistance to language is pain's peculiar grammatical relationship with the external world. Whereas other emotional, perceptual, and somatic states take objects (for example, we speak of being in love with *your partner,* listening to *the radio,* hungry for *pie*), enabling us to move beyond the body and into a shared world, pain does not. Consequently, the pain sufferer is deprived of a grammatical bridge from the alienating world of intense pain. Pain, for Scarry, destroys language and worlds.[53]

Despite these challenges, two principal claims that I explore in this book are that pain is not as private and unsharable as is often assumed, and that language and other expressive modes constitute important resources for bringing pain out of the private realm. To open up these claims, it is first important to consider what we mean by the "sharability" of pain. For Scarry, and others who use her argument, pain experience cannot be shared because it can only be partially (and hence, incompletely) objectified through language. Thus, Scarry concludes, "Whatever pain achieves, it achieves in part through its unsharability, and it ensures this unsharability through its resistance to language."[54]

Yet objectification through language is not the only sense in which we might think of pain being shared. In making this claim, I join scholars such as the anthropologists Veena Das and Talal Asad and the historian Julie Livingston, who have questioned whether it makes sense to locate pain solely in individual bodies.[55] They suggest that, more than being an embodied experience separate from the social world, pain itself is always already culturally constituted. My own contribution to this line of thinking is to consider the ways in which pain might be shared through practices of care and expressive modes. Veena Das suggests that saying "I am in pain" is not only a statement of fact but also a plea for acknowledgement.[56] "Pain, in this rendering," Das writes, "is not that inexpressible something that destroys communication or marks an exit from one's existence in language. Instead, it makes a claim asking for acknowledgment, which may be given or denied. In either case, it is not a referential statement that is simply pointing to an inner object."[57] Thus, for Das, pain is not shared by creating an externalized representation of an internal state that is made comprehensible through this projection. Rather, sharing is constituted through social action—in this case, a claim for acknowledging another person's pain. This view of sharing pain hinges on a performative view of language: the idea that *saying* is also a form of *doing*.[58]

My understanding of the social dimensions of pain aligns with this broader orientation to the possibilities of shared pain. Approaching pain in this way enables us to situate a putative private experience within an intersubjective milieu and to understand how both experiencing and responding to pain is a deeply relational enterprise. Furthermore, I understand the explanation of pain to be fundamentally at stake in the plea for acknowledgment alluded to above. The person in pain cries out for an explanation for her suffering, and the language of medicine offers one grammatical framework for responding to this call.[59]

### Explanatory Roadblocks

If chronic pain represents a failure of medicine, as several analysts have suggested,[60] then this failure can be read partially as a failure of explanation. In thinking about such failures, it may be helpful to revisit the four dimensions of biomedical explanation that I introduced in the previous section. First, *cause*. From a biomedical perspective, explaining pain is closely related to diagnostic nosology. Yet the etiological mechanisms for pain are complex, and there may not be a simple linear relationship between pain and underlying pathology. As with many medical conditions, causal explanations for pain may be located at various (and across multiple) levels, including the individual body, the family system, and the larger social structure. The application of these various explanatory frameworks hinges in turn on whether we understand pain primarily through the lens of biology, as in sickle cell disease;[61] psychodynamic theory, as in the case of hysteria;[62] or the wider political economy, as in what Nicaraguan women call *dolor de cerebro* ("brain ache").[63]

Biomedical practitioners have amassed a large number of labels for pain that does not have an identifiable pathophysiological cause, from *inorganic* to *functional,* while *psychogenic* and *psychosomatic* pain point more specifically to psychological causes. Likewise, a wide body of clinical and anthropological literature has examined the concept of *somatization,* the notion that bodily pain may serve as a medium for communicating social and emotional troubles that escape verbal channels.[64] Other terms, such as *intractable,* convey that pain has not responded to standard treatment. These terms all point, in various ways, to the failures of biomedicine: failures to explain adequately why pain has occurred and to respond adequately to its presence.

*Certainty* is the second dimension of biomedical explanation identified previously. While uncertainty is endemic across medical settings, the uncertainty inherent in pain explanations is of a very particular sort. Whereas much medical uncertainty crystallizes around epistemological questions—for example, how physicians can know what will prove the best course of treatment—pain clinicians must grapple with *ontological* uncertainty: that is, uncertainty about whether a person is truly in pain and the nature of pain itself. This brings us to *truth*, the third dimension in this typology. The inability to read the body for signs of certainty and truth constitutes a major failure of biomedicine's treatment of pain.

Finally, explanations of pain traffic in issues of *meaning*. Fundamentally, to explain pain is to endow it with meaning, providing a sense of what one is suffering *for*, as opposed to what the philosopher Emmanuel Lévinas calls "useless" suffering.[65] The mid-twentieth-century American anesthesiologist Henry Beecher observed that soldiers wounded during World War II reported pain less frequently than would be expected and proposed that this was because their injuries had been sustained while engaged in honorable pursuits.[66] Similarly, the context of childbirth may make the intense pain that accompanies it seem somewhat less excruciating. In certain cultural and historical settings, pain has likewise occupied a role in artistic expression, ritual, and initiations.[67] In contrast to these examples, as I describe in more detail below, biomedical concerns about what chronic pain is *for*, both biologically and morally, have emerged rather recently. From a contemporary biomedical perspective, the essential value of diagnostic labels lies in the meanings that they have for the practitioners who bestow and the patients who receive them. From this perspective, unexplained pain is a biomedical failure, because it has no meaning.

## THE SOCIAL LIFE OF PAIN

However solitary the experience of pain might be, chronic pain treatment is a fundamentally social enterprise that draws on the expertise of a range of clinical actors, as well as the cooperative involvement of patients, families, and friends. Elaine Scarry may be correct that pain destroys worlds, yet it also creates them anew, since networks of clinicians and loved ones form to care for those afflicted.[68] Cassandra Grindall was treated in the West Clinic not only by Dr. Novak, a physician board-certified in pediatric pain and adolescent medicine, but also by Ted Bridgewater, the clinic's acupuncturist, Rebecca Hunter, the clinic's child and family therapist, and Charlotte LeFevre, the clinic's hypnotherapist. Each week, over the course of Cassandra's treatment, these clinicians gathered around a conference table along with several other colleagues, staff members, students, and observers to discuss Cassandra's progress and treatment plan, along with those of many other clinic patients.

Multidisciplinary pain clinics like the West Clinic were popularized in the United States in the 1960s. The anesthesiologist John Bonica introduced the concept of the pain clinic by bringing together clinicians from different specialties to care for patients as a team.[69] Scientific advances in understanding the roles of learning, memory, and attention in physiological pain mechanisms helped to justify the use of psychosocial therapies in addition to medication and surgical intervention, affirming the role of a multidisciplinary therapeutic approach. Anthropological research during this era also generated a growing awareness of the relationship between culture and pain by documenting variation in how people from various ethnic groups respond to and express pain.[70] Together, these innovations helped to usher new concerns with the social into the treatment arena.

Many contemporary pain clinics, including the West Clinic, subscribe to the biopsychosocial model of disease introduced by the psychiatrist George Engel in the late 1970s.[71] Where the biomedical model tends to characterize diseases as either somatic or mental, leaving little room for interactions between the two domains, Engel drew on systems theory to argue for a new medical model that would account for dynamic interactions between individual psychology, behavior, sociocultural contexts, and biological processes. Although it has since been the target of incisive critiques from social scientists and psychiatrists for disregarding the structural determinants of health,[72] this framework has become dominant, even hegemonic, in pain medicine, ensuring a role for multidisciplinary treatment.

The growth of multidisciplinary pain clinics in the decades following Bonica's pioneering efforts was accompanied by the transformation of pain from a *symptom* of disease to a disease in its own right.[73] Where once, in our evolutionary history, pain tended to serve a purpose—to warn of the danger of touching fire, for instance, or to signal an injury that needed attention—chronic pain has lost this biological signaling function. Designating chronic pain as a distinct clinical category created a need for a specific assemblage of experts and therapeutic practices to manage and treat it. (What actually constitutes chronic pain is a matter of some debate, though experts generally agree that pain should last three to six months before it is considered chronic.)[74]

A defining feature of contemporary multidisciplinary pain treatment is a shift in orientation from curing pain to managing its effects. The elimination of pain is rarely an expressed goal of multidisciplinary pain treatment; instead, treatment is aimed at improving day-to-day "functioning" through a range of behavioral, psychosocial, and pharmaceutical strategies.[75] Consequently, multidisciplinary pain clinics have often been characterized as "the end of the road"[76] or "the end of the line"[77] insofar as they signal a recalibration of expectations regarding the ends of treatment.

A close look at multidisciplinary pain clinics reveals myriad ways in which pain, that ostensibly private phenomenon, enters the social realm. Socialization and learning have played an important role in the design and organization of these clinics since their inception. Drawing on the behavioral paradigms dominant in contemporary clinical psychology, a primary goal of Western biomedical pain treatment has been to "resocialize" patients to manage their pain better.[78] Inpatient pain clinics, for example, rely on the assumption that patients will learn effective pain management strategies from "model" patients, while calibrating the behavioral expression of pain is vital to the kind of care that patients receive and to whether their pain is taken seriously.[79] Relational goals, such as helping patients resume work and family responsibilities, have also been a key component of multidisciplinary pain treatment, reinforcing expectations for a particular way of responding to chronic pain.[80] Such program characteristics highlight the ways in which rehabilitation is predicated on particular notions of ideal personhood, suggesting that it is not only the failure of biomedicine that is at stake in chronic pain management, but also the failure of *persons* to abide by specific moral worldviews.

Today, pain medicine has become a booming industry in the United States. In hospitals and clinics across the country, pain is now a distinct medical subspecialty, encompassing services from routine surgical anesthesiology and pharmaceutical management to spinal blocks and end-of-life palliation. Recent estimates suggest that approximately a hundred million Americans live with chronic pain conditions, resulting in costs of $560–635 billion per year in medical treatment and lost productivity. And, while pain has historically been underfunded in the U.S. biomedical research complex, in part because none of the branches of the National Institutes of Health are specifically devoted to it, a 2011 report of the Institute of Medicine acknowledged the need for greater research funding and put pain on the map as a national public health priority.[81]

Pain medicine has also left its imprint on American society more broadly. The historian of medicine Keith Wailoo has documented the complex moral and political economies that have shaped political and legal responses to pain and disability since World War II, arguing that pain has served as a battleground for contestation over liberal and conservative political perspectives, as exemplified by debates about the government's role in supporting people with disabilities.[82] More recently, pervasive anxieties about the "epidemic" of prescription painkiller abuse have cut across class lines to infiltrate the popular imaginary.[83] Such effects highlight the ways in which pain far outstrips facile distinctions between public and private. As we will see, pain reverberates through households and communities in ways that belie its frequent characterization as solitary and private.

### Situating Pediatric Pain

In the United States, pediatric pain medicine is located in the realm of tertiary care, medical services performed by physicians with specialized training. Pediatric pain clinics are generally situated in hospital settings, and often, though not always, in academic medical centers. Children and adolescents are typically referred to pediatric pain experts by pediatricians or, more frequently, other pediatric subspecialists, such as gastroenterologists, orthopedists, rheumatologists, and neurologists. These hierarchies of referral, in combination with the insurance restrictions and expensive co-pays often imposed on tertiary care, mean that pediatric pain treatment may be somewhat more difficult for lower-income patients to obtain.

Pediatric pain clinics tend to occupy a precarious status in the US hospital infrastructure because tertiary care clinics continue to rely on a fee-for-service reimbursement model, in which a clinic's income depends on the number of tests ordered and interventions performed.[84] Pediatric pain clinics, however, generally offer few interventions, relying more heavily on psychological, behavioral, and complementary/alternative therapeutic strategies, all of which bring in less income from patients' insurance companies. As one U.S.-based pediatric pain physician told me, "There's inadequate reimbursement for pain management in general. So our pain management service loses money and we have to rely upon the largesse of our hospital to keep us going year after year." Consequently, many clinicians I met during my fieldwork worried about their clinics' long-term security. Many subsidized clinical work with funding from research grants. One Canadian clinician with whom I spoke noted that many clinics faced a difficult dilemma: while they were not getting all of the referrals they should be to help kids who are in pain, they could not accommodate any more patients than they already had due to their limited clinic hours.

There was one important exception to this general trend: pediatric clinics that employed anesthesiologists (unlike the West Clinic) enjoyed relatively more financial security. As one psychologist explained to me, "Because our two physicians are in the OR [operating room] the rest of the time . . . they make money through the rest of their activities. And so, our clinic does not make money, but we've also not been scrutinized [by hospital administrators] over that." This particular point runs counter to the stereotype that anesthesiologists are motivated by a desire to make a lot of money without working very hard. At least in the field of pediatric pain, many anesthesiologists continue to assist in surgical procedures so that they can have more freedom to offer care that is less well compensated.

An additional reason why pediatric pain treatment is especially challenging is because of high rates of psychiatric co-morbidity, particularly anxiety and depression.[85] Dr. Novak once remarked that her patients were more psychiatrically complex than those of any mental health clinic. To some extent, then, the institutional challenges of pediatric pain management reflect the chronic underfunding of mental health care in the United States more generally—although American children and adolescents have a somewhat easier time obtaining treatment for mental health issues than do adults.[86] The high rates of emotional symptoms in pediatric pain patients also reflect long-standing questions about psychological causality in chronic pain and how we configure, and continually renegotiate, the relationship between body and mind.

For adolescents, these questions take on new urgency when heightened by the challenges of what can often be an emotionally difficult time. As we will see, patients in the West Clinic faced a range of stressors: pressure to perform well academically while juggling multiple extracurricular demands, the sometimes impractical desire of getting into an elite college, turbulent friendships, bullying, unrequited young love, or the threat of unraveling kinship ties due to fighting in the household. To be sure, the contours these pressures were marked by the West Clinic patients' privileged social position. What interests me in this book is how these pressures became taken up, ignored, or rejected in explanations of pain, and particularly how they interlaced with—and challenged—neurobiological understandings of pain.

## THE WEST CLINIC

The West Clinic's senior physician was Dr. Novak, an accomplished yet unassuming woman in her sixties. She trained in pediatrics and adolescent medicine before starting the pain program in the 1990s to care for children and adolescents with complicated pain conditions. Dr. Novak had recruited Dr. Petrosian to join the clinic several years before my research began. At the time, Dr. Petrosian was in his early thirties and completing a fellowship in a different pediatric subspecialty. Following his fellowship, he split his time between the West Clinic and his own private clinic. Unlike Dr. Novak, Dr. Petrosian was not board-certified in pediatric pain, but he had learned from Dr. Novak over the years that they worked together.

The clinic did not offer surgical interventions or diagnostic tests, which patients typically underwent in other pediatric subspecialty clinics (e.g., gastroenterology, neurology, and orthopedics) prior to being referred there. The primary treatment that Dr. Novak and Dr. Petrosian offered was pharmaceutical, although Dr. Petrosian sometimes performed trigger-point injections.[87] There was no inpatient pain service associated with the West Clinic, but patients were occasionally referred to a pain program in another part of the state for inpatient treatment.

In these respects, the West Clinic was similar to many other pediatric pain clinics internationally, within which multidisciplinary and noninterventionist approaches have been widely adopted. Where the West Clinic stood out, however, was in its setup and internal organization. Aside from Dr. Novak and Dr. Petrosian, who saw patients in a weekly outpatient clinic in the pediatric wing of a tertiary-care hospital, the rest of the multidisciplinary pain team saw patients in their private practices, which were located throughout the community. The team only met in the hospital on a weekly basis to discuss patient progress and coordinate treatment plans. In this sense, the pain team functioned more as a loose consortium than as a formal hospital division.

This idiosyncratic organizational structure reflects certain bureaucratic limits on institutionalizing pain. In part, this is because pain appears to belong both everywhere and nowhere: just as chronic pain may resist localization in the body (for example, to a specific organ system), it may also resist localization within the American medical system (to a specific hospital division). It is also because pediatric pain medicine, and particularly the West Clinic's holistic and integrative medical approach, is not especially lucrative. Insurance companies pay much less for physicians' counsel than they do for high-tech interventions and tests. During the time of my research, the clinic faced increasing financial pressure from hospital administrators to bring in more money.

A major part of Dr. Novak and Dr. Petrosian's clinical responsibilities entailed overseeing referrals to clinicians on the multidisciplinary team, which included a psychiatrist, two psychologists, a family therapist, two physical therapists, an acupuncturist, a music therapist, an art therapist, a craniosacral therapist, a hypnotherapist, and a yoga instructor. Dr. Novak had assembled the pain team through her professional network and personal contacts in the community. Some of the clinicians she had approached following the recommendations of friends or colleagues, while others she recruited after receiving their therapeutic services herself, as with Tess Bergman, the yoga teacher, who helped Dr. Novak rehabilitate from a difficult surgery. Occasionally, a clinician joined the team after pursuing Dr. Novak directly, as was the case with Craig Davies, the craniosacral therapist.[88] Many of the clinicians had not worked with pediatric pain populations prior to their involvement in the West Clinic, but were lured into the work by Dr. Novak's holistic approach to integrative care. As a team, the clinicians were committed to an ethos of collegiality, teamwork, and harmony. They maintained this through frequent e-mail and phone contact, annual retreats, and weekly hour-long team meetings, which provided a forum for prioritizing treatment goals and resolving concerns about specific patients.

The West Clinic treated patients as young as five and occasionally as old as twenty-five. The majority of patients, however, and the group that I chose to focus my research on, were adolescents between the ages of eleven and eighteen. Generally speaking, referrals for an individual patient were limited to two or three members of the team, although in some cases, patients saw as many as five or more clinicians. Referral decisions were made at the end of an initial two-hour consultation and reflected an attempt to balance several factors. First, many families drove up to two or three hours to visit the West Clinic, and several families traveled from out of state during the course of my study. For these families, weekly therapy appointments with members of the pain team were obviously a problem. Yet even for families who lived within thirty miles of the clinic, the notorious freeway traffic in Southern California sometimes made therapy appointments an all-day affair, which could be quite taxing. For this reason, the patient's extracurricular activities and the family's schedule also factored into the number and type of referrals made.

Financial considerations were also important, because most of the team's services were not covered by medical insurance and families varied in their ability to pay for them. Most U.S. insurance companies provide coverage for a limited number of physical therapy sessions, and many cover acupuncture treatment. Neither the psychiatrist, Dr. Sterling, nor any of the psychologists accepted insurance, but some families were able to get a modest portion of their fees reimbursed by their insurance companies. Beyond acupuncture, most complementary and alternative medical (CAM) therapies were not reimbursed, and families were expected to pay out of pocket. Consequently, the West Clinic served a predominantly middle- to upper-class population. Sometimes, Dr. Novak or Dr. Petrosian asked directly whether the family could afford CAM therapies, but often judgments about the family's finances were made based on information about where they lived, how the parents were employed, and whether the patients attended public or private school. While sometimes accurate, such demographic judgments could also prove to be crude sociological tools for diagnosing families' economic health. Moreover, some families did not feel comfortable expressing their financial limitations. In one case, it was several months into a patient's treatment before the team learned that her father was unemployed and had not yet been paid for a job he had recently finished.

Finally, Dr. Novak and Dr. Petrosian also attempted to balance referrals between specific therapeutic modalities that were perceived to offer similar benefits. For example, it was unlikely that a patient would be referred to both hypnotherapy and biofeedback, which both targeted the mind as a mechanism for pain control, or physical therapy and yoga, which both aimed to develop the patient's strength and flexibility. Similarly, because the art therapist also had a psychology degree, it was unlikely for a patient to be referred to art therapy in addition to individual psychotherapy. Certain therapies were also considered to be particularly effective for specific diagnoses, such as acupuncture for headaches and irritable bowel syndrome. Psychology and physical therapy referrals were determined largely by geography, because the team contained multiple psychologists and physical therapists whose offices were located in different parts of the broader metropolitan region. While not absolute rules, these guidelines helped to ensure a mostly smooth division of therapeutic labor.

After the first clinic appointment, most patients saw their primary physician every four weeks at the beginning, and then less frequently once their pain was under control. In general, the better they were doing, the less often they came to see Dr. Novak or Dr. Petrosian in the outpatient clinic, which met one day per week. How often patients saw the rest of the clinicians depended on the nature of the pain problem and the family's resources. Most clinicians hoped to see patients on a weekly basis under ideal circumstances, and some clinicians requested a certain number of sessions as a minimum. However, treatment plans were largely individualized based on the patient's and family's needs.

The clinicians prided themselves on their carefully orchestrated treatment plans and commitment to frequent communication with families. Family contact was largely handled with painstaking care, which tended to set the West Clinic apart from other clinical settings that patients and families had experience in. Although they did not think of themselves as offering luxury or "concierge" medicine, the West Clinic did offer a standard of care that went far beyond what was typical, even for tertiary-care clinics.[89] As Dr. Petrosian acknowledged, speaking to me about his division of time between the West Clinic and his own private clinic, "at 20 percent commitment, it's more like a 40–45 percent commitment. 'Cause they're paging you at any time during the weekend. Checking e-mails. We've really made it concierge service without the price."

In addition to fielding questions and concerns between clinic appointments, clinicians stepped in when needed to speak with educators, advocating for their patients in a variety of nonmedical contexts. Rebecca Hunter often telephoned school administrators to ask them to permit patients to return to school bit by bit after a long-term absence, for example, by starting with lunchtime. Dr. Novak occasionally became involved in legal matters, as with a patient's custody battle during her parents' divorce. On at least one occasion, she visited a patient at home who was having great difficulty getting out of bed. Clinic staff also triaged communication with other physicians caring for their patients to ensure that everyone stayed in the loop. Families were, for the most part, extraordinarily grateful for such extra care, but a few appeared to test the limits of the clinicians' goodwill.

Any illusions of luxury medicine must also be tempered by the broader conditions of constraint within which the West Clinic operated. Financially, the end of 2008 and beginning of 2009 was a difficult time for many Americans, and the families in my study were no exception. By the fall of 2008, when the subprime mortgage crisis had come to a head, the banking system had all but collapsed, and unemployment rates reached new lows, it was widely accepted that the United States had entered the worst financial crisis since the Great Depression. Amid this rapid economic decline, medical treatment for complex pain problems and associated psychological care might easily be construed as luxury items that many families simply could no longer afford.

One day, in November 2008, Arlene Weiss, one of the West Clinic's clinical psychologists, mentioned at the end of a team meeting that one of her patients was no longer able to come to therapy because her parents could not afford it. "They're actually worried about even keeping their house at this point," Arlene explained. She was down to almost no patients, and wondered if anyone else on the team was experiencing similar problems. Rebecca Hunter was in the same position; no one could afford psychotherapy. These admissions were met with a grave silence, which I found alarming. Typically, the clinicians were quick to jump in with a comment or suggestion. Several clinicians had in fact told me privately that certain people on the team were a little too quick to offer judgments or advice. The silence in this case was incongruous and unnerving.

Dr. Novak tried to buffer families from the impact of the economic recession, volunteering to have the clinical coordinator, Nina Herrera, write to insurance companies advocating for the coverage of CAM therapies. However, this strategy was not often effective, and it typically demanded a lot of follow-up attention from families. In one notable case, Kaiser Permanente, an HMO insurance company,[90] approved eight sessions with Charlotte LeFevre because there were no pediatric pain clinicians in its network. However, this approval was only granted following the persistent advocacy of the patient's mother over a two-month period and a thick stack of paperwork completed by Nina and Charlotte. Cases like this proved the exception rather than the rule.

The clinicians worked to find creative solutions for families in need, lowering fees, tapping into free resources such as school counselors and university research studies that might offer short-term psychotherapeutic services free of charge, and, when necessary, privileging physical therapy and acupuncture, which held some hope of insurance reimbursement, over other therapeutic modalities. In one notable case, Rebecca Hunter, much to her husband's dismay, held onto hundreds of dollars in un-cashed checks because of a family's financial insecurity. Rebecca knew that cashing the checks would cause stress for the parents, which would likely have a negative effect on her young patient. After several months, Rebecca finally ripped up the checks and submitted the therapy sessions as a tax write-off.

The clinic's efforts to accommodate families experiencing economic hardship ran counter to competing pressures from hospital administrators, however. As the economy worsened, the West Clinic became vulnerable within the broader hospital structure because it was not as profitable as other clinics, and Dr. Novak was forced to subsidize administrative support through her research grants. As Tess Bergman put it, "We don't have a space, we don't have money, we see people once a week, you know. I think you can't really get [a] fully functioning, great program going under those circumstances. . . . It's not really set up in a way that's helpful for the families."

One particularly evocative example of the tension between accommodating families and bowing to hospital financial pressures concerned Dr. Novak's short-lived attempts to change the clinic's e-mail policy. Most clinicians on the pain team prided themselves on being easily accessible by e-mail but, as Dr. Novak noted at a meeting in September 2008, this took up clinicians' valuable time without compensation. She urged the team to limit e-mail contact and encourage parents to schedule appointments instead. The requested change never quite caught on—in large part because the clinicians did not seem to mind the extra e-mails and did not want to deprive their patients of this privileged mode of communication. Yet its incongruity with the clinic's overriding ethos of care highlighted the paradoxes within which Dr. Novak was operating. In her day-to-day practice, responsibilities to patients and to institutional administrators were systematically at odds, pitting the clinic's economy of care against its underlying ethos.

. . .

While the West Clinic treated some patients with chronic pain resulting from diseases like cancer and sickle cell disease, most of its patients suffered from pain with poorly understood etiology. Because *All in Your Head* is a book about the language of pain, I have thought carefully about the terms employed to characterize pain. Common clinical labels such as *functional* and *intractable* are problematic, insofar as they can contribute to the delegitimization of pain that medical practitioners cannot explain and make patients with these conditions seem less worthy of clinical attention. Furthermore, social scientists may unintentionally collude in a disavowal of the psychological dimensions of puzzling symptoms by adopting such terminology.[91] With these caveats in mind, I will simply say that this book focuses on chronic pain conditions that lacked a clear-cut etiology and baffled patients and practitioners alike, such as chronic daily headaches and recurrent abdominal pain.

Despite the tremendous amount of ambiguity inherent in such symptomatology, the clinicians worked explicitly to legitimize all pain as real, to offset the stigma that chronic pain patients have historically encountered. Accordingly, clinical discourse relied heavily on neurobiological language, particularly in early encounters with patients and their families. Neurobiological explanatory tropes cast pain as a real illness, rendering patients worthy of clinical attention. At times, however, this language came up hard against ingrained cultural models of mind and body, which tend to suggest that the mind is to blame for pain that lacks an identifiable organic cause.[92] Moreover, while the clinicians made clear that they did not believe that pain was "all in your head" they did expect patients to take significant responsibility for their care and pain management. This clear distinction between causal responsibility and responsible self-care occasionally produced confusion for patients and families, tracking pathways of blame.

The West Clinic's rhetorical emphasis on legitimizing all pain did not preclude clinicians from holding private opinions about the reality of patients' pain complaints. Tess Bergman left a powerful impression on me when I asked her whether yoga worked better for certain kinds of pain. "Well, I think it works best when it's real," she replied. "You know, like, it works best for people who have a real problem." When I pressed her further to explain what she meant, she backed away uneasily, though she did acknowledge, later in our interview, that she particularly liked treating patients with conditions such as rheumatoid arthritis and lupus.

Tess's comment is all the more striking in light of the West Clinic's commitment to treating all pain as if it were, in fact, real, when speaking to patients and families. This commitment illustrates the clinic's moral stance toward affirming the authenticity of adolescents' suffering. Yet what might be at stake if the pain were not real, and why would clinicians work so hard to legitimize it? I propose that "unreal" pain would suggest deeper troubles, which biomedicine might not be equipped to address. Upholding the reality of pain was therefore a gesture of care aimed at shielding families from their children's vulnerability and preserving cultural ideals of childhood innocence.

### ETHICS AND METHOD IN CLINICAL ETHNOGRAPHY

One Sunday afternoon, I went to the home of Mark Siegel, a fourteen-year-old boy who had been suffering from chronic regional pain syndrome (CRPS) in his arm for over a year.[93] Greeting me at the door, Mark's mother, Julie, explained that she works in the health-care field and was eager to help with my research. While these motives certainly seemed innocuous enough, I became uneasy when, during the course of the interview, Julie asked me to reassure her multiple times that the West Clinic could help her son. It was, as I noted in my field notes that evening, "a tricky position to be in because I did not want to dash her hopes, and yet I also did not want to be held responsible in any way if the visit proved unsuccessful. I ended up saying that most kids do have some improvement."[94]

My initial encounter with Julie prompted me to think about the ethical entanglements of medical anthropologists in clinical settings, wherein patients and families may be apt to pin their hopes for treatment on the research relationship. Over the course of Mark's treatment, it became clear to me that, far from a purely altruistic desire to help the advancement of medicine, Julie (quite understandably) brought her own agenda to my research. This included her expectation that I would relay back to the pain team how committed she was to her son, and how invested the family was in his treatment. It also included, on different occasions, more explicit bids for assistance: to help secure a phone call back from a clinician who had not responded to her messages, or, much later, to relay information about a treatment that Mark obtained outside of the West Clinic to other clinic patients (the latter of which I refused).[95]

As with any sort of anthropological fieldwork, clinical ethnography—a domain of anthropological scholarship that is principally concerned with unpacking the cultural logic of clinical practices[96]—contains specific ethical and methodological challenges that are very much intertwined. Elsewhere, I have written about the difficulties of positioning oneself as an independent researcher—that is, one who is not employed by or directly affiliated with a clinic—when one recruits participants from a clinic population, since a clinical tie of some sort is necessary to facilitate this sort of research.[97] Consequently, conducting anthropological research in clinical settings comes with certain practical entailments in which patients may harbor misunderstandings about the relationship between research participation and the quality of their care. In interviews, families often referred to their experiences in the West Clinic with descriptors such as "you guys," which conveyed their implicit assumptions that I was part of the clinic's staff. Like Julie Siegel, they sometimes expected that I would relay information back to members of the pain team about how much their child was suffering or how hard they were working therapeutically.

Maintaining a critical gaze on both clinical and family settings created an additional layer of methodological complexity for me, because I had to tack back and forth between opposing perspectives and alignments. Such ethnographic positioning created an ethical challenge, requiring me to bracket my sympathies continuously in an effort to understand what was at stake for actors in different encounters. This sometimes meant understanding that a physician might have lost patience with a family because the clinic day was long and there were always too many patients to see, or that a "difficult" mother was only yelling at a staff member because she was anxious, helpless, and tired. While I have strived to maintain a balance between aligning with the disparate perspectives of families and clinicians, I acknowledge the possibility of misrecognition.

. . .

The research for this book involved a variety of ethnographic activities that I carried out over eighteen months in 2008–9. Most of my data resulted from observations of patient encounters and West Clinic team meetings and interviews with seventy-six patients, parents, and clinicians about their experiences living with, managing, and treating pediatric pain.[98] I also collected longitudinal video recordings of four focal families in a range of family, biomedical, and complementary and alternative therapeutic settings during five to ten months of treatment.[99] Finally, in order to explore the culture of pediatric pain management beyond the specific institutional setting I was studying, I attended two professional pain conferences. At both of these conferences, I interviewed several physicians and psychologists from the United States, Canada, and Western Europe.

In order to get a sense of how the clinical styles of the two physicians differed, I took turns observing Dr. Novak and Dr. Petrosian in the West Clinic. I arranged my time so that I could follow particular patients longitudinally. Before I observed new patients in intake appointments, the physician approached the family and explained my study, asking permission for me to speak with them. If the family agreed, I introduced myself and the goals of my research, and obtained the family's consent for me to observe the consultation. Often, I was not the only outside observer, since the physicians were frequently "shadowed" by medical students, residents, or even pre-med undergraduates, and occasionally by physicians from other hospitals interested in learning about pediatric pain management—a fact that partially accounts for the ease with which I was able to gain access to this highly intimate clinical setting. As a result, and also because multiple family members accompanied some patients to the clinic, the examination rooms were often crowded. I practiced slinking into narrow corners and leaning against walls unobtrusively, trying not to get in the way. I did carry a clipboard and take notes, but this did not make me stand out, since most of the others in the room (including the families) were also taking notes.

During patient consultations, I usually remained silent, but if the physician (and his or her entourage) left the room to talk about the treatment plan or to retrieve a prescription pad, I would often remain behind to talk to the family. Many parents were intrigued to find out just what an anthropologist was doing in a hospital and asked questions about my research. At the end of the visit, I asked if families would be willing to be contacted by phone in the future. Many of the families I encountered this way I interviewed later in the study. At team meetings, I limited my notes to a few essential key words and wrote more detailed summaries of what was discussed immediately afterward.

· The families I interviewed were mostly, although not exclusively, white, and came largely from middle- to upper-class backgrounds. Two-thirds of the patients I interviewed had been in pain for more than six months before their first clinic visit. Almost half were not attending school regularly at the time of clinic enrollment. In many cases, these adolescents had enrolled in a home-schooling program, but some were too sick to do even this.

. . .

As will become clear in the pages that follow, the fieldwork on which this book is based raises several challenges for ethnographic representation, particularly questions of generalizability. Much of what initially captured my attention in the early days of my research was how unusual the West Clinic seemed within the broader landscape of US healthcare. The clinic's patient population represented the upper end of the socioeconomic spectrum. Apart from serving a large number of Jewish families, it hardly reflected the surrounding area's ethnic and racial diversity. The dispersal of clinical sites, diffuse structure, and limited reimbursement for many therapies likewise distinguished it from other pediatric pain clinics in which I interviewed clinicians. Beyond these demographic and organizational characteristics, the clinical discourse and explanatory models that I encountered in the West Clinic were also quite exceptional. In early presentations of my research, scholarly audiences seemed almost transfixed by the clinic's distinctive language and metaphors. While it was certainly encouraging when others found my work interesting, it also made it difficult, at times, to move beyond the data and get to bigger questions and claims.

Particularity is not usually a detriment for the anthropologist ethnographer, since we do not typically worry about generalizability writ large. Much to the contrary, particularity has long been touted as one of the hallmark features of ethnographic fieldwork.[100] And yet the suggestion of idiosyncrasy raises questions about intellectual relevance and intelligibility, about how to enter into conversation with a wider community of scholars. Even in anthropology, there can be a certain cynicism regarding scholarly work that appears to be "merely" a case study.[101] At best, such reservations reveal doubts about whether a case can find a pathway—a language, a set of relationships—that enable an escape from its own interiority; at worst, such reservations express fear of an ethnographic solipsism that threatens to make the research irrelevant.

These are real worries, which I have spent many anxious hours mulling over while working on this book.[102] In responding to these concerns, I have been greatly inspired by Julie Livingston's invitation to think of the clinic as a microcosm: "an instantiation of," yet "only one possibility."[103] Livingston's beautiful ethnography of an oncology ward in Botswana shows that probing a single clinical site in all of its particularities can offer an opening onto larger cultural and historical processes. As the literary critic Lauren Berlant has written, "To ask the question of what makes something a case, and not merely a gestural instance, illustration, or example, is to query the adequacy of an object to bear the weight of an example worthy of attending to and taking a lesson from."[104]

In this spirit, the lessons of my ethnographic case are twofold. First, the West Clinic stands as a microcosm of interpretation and explanation at times when the brute force of pain telescopes one's world and overwhelms one's sense-making faculties. Second, the pain and suffering found there offer a microcosm of the kinds of struggles facing many American families today and the intimacy and care with which they face them. As the anthropologist Jean Jackson has put it, in her work on chronic pain, "the best locations for understanding a society are the sites where things don't work."[105] It should be clear from this that I do not claim that this ethnographic case will stand as a microcosm for pediatric pain medicine, or even pediatric pain medicine in the United States. Rather, the experiences and therapeutic processes that I documented reflect something far more basic about the ways in which contemporary Americans understand, translate, and manage distress—concerns that, I hope, will bear the weight of your attention.

## SUMMARY OF CHAPTERS

*All in Your Head* is organized around three prevailing explanatory frames—neurobiology, psychodynamics, and societal stress—which form the focus of successive chapters. The chapters examine how each of these frames provide conceptual tools for making sense of pain. Chapter 1 begins by describing how families make their way to specialized pediatric pain clinics, a journey that lands them, as one physician put it, "at the bottom of the funnel": spun around, siphoned through a narrowing range of treatment options, and spit out the bottom with nowhere else to go. Taking the funnel as a point of departure, I explore the metaphors that pediatric pain practitioners use to explain chronic pain to adolescents and families.

Having established that metaphors are a key element of clinical rhetoric, I turn to the question of *how* they persuade by examining how explanations of pain take shape within the clinical encounter. In chapter 2, the first of two chapters that focus on the neurobiological explanatory frame, I examine a clinical explanatory model that linked the neurobiology of chronic pain to certain qualities of smart, talented, and virtuous adolescents. As Dr. Novak put it, there was something about "the neurobiology of being smart" that made these adolescents more susceptible to pain problems. Drawing on close analysis of video-recorded clinical interactions, I illustrate how this explanatory model and its constituent metaphors (e.g., "smart neurons") transformed the meaning of pain by depicting patients in a morally favorable manner. In doing so, it laid the groundwork from the first clinical meeting for a particular ethic of clinical care that emphasized the patient's personal responsibility for treatment.

In chapter 3, I explore a local explanatory model that held that some patients developed chronic pain because their brains were "sticky." Clinicians used terms such as "sticky brains" and "sticky neurons" to describe the perseverative thoughts and quirky behavior that characterized a sizable minority of the program's chronic pain patients who were believed to show signs of pervasive developmental disorders and, consequently, did not respond well to treatment. The discourse on sticky brains dramatically altered the meaning of chronic pain by suggesting that a preexisting psychological disorder was responsible for the patient's failure to respond to standard treatment. Yet invoking the brain (and not, for example, the mind or head) in diagnostic reasoning asserts a different sort of ontological claim on the presence of pain than declaring it, more dubiously, "all in your head." The term "sticky brains" thus encapsulates some of the core tensions—between biological and psychological, psyche and soma, real and "unreal" symptoms—wrapped up in explanations of pain.

Although clinicians characterized chronic pain as a neurobiological problem in initial conversations with patients and families, they often privately attributed intractable pain to pathological family ties and targeted parents as a key site of intervention and blame. Chapter 4 explores how neurobiological and psychodynamic explanatory frames were stitched together over time. I focus especially on the West Clinic's team meetings as a site of negotiation of blame to illustrate how different explanations took shape in what I refer to as "backstage" and "onstage" clinical spaces. Focusing on a single case, I trace the causal pathways that clinicians drew between family psychodynamics and a fourteen-year-old patient's mysterious symptoms. By highlighting the assumptions about family life that influenced the team's approach to treatment, I show that treatment was aimed, not only at managing pain, but also at prescribing moral and cultural worldviews vis-à-vis adolescent development, family roles, and desirable parenting practices.

Finally, chapter 5 considers societal stress as an explanatory frame for pain. The idea that chronic pain might be caused by societal distress has its roots in a long line of cultural and historical narratives that have linked illness to rapid social change and the pressures of modernity. After reviewing this body of work, I situate the experience of West Clinic patients within a larger conversation about American adolescence and the culture of stress, particularly vis-à-vis the pressures of achievement-oriented high schools in middle- and upper-middle class communities. I argue that for some adolescents, chronic patienthood offered a pathway out of a stressful life and a welcome opportunity to reimagine aspirational futures.

In the concluding chapter, I take a step back to articulate why explanations matter in the biomedical realm. Having demonstrated the rich and varied potential of explanatory frameworks for pain, I discuss how my findings challenge the view that biomedicine depends on a referential view of language. Explanations matter, I ultimately argue, because textual representations have the power to transform the body in pain and experiences of illness. Moreover, contrary to social scientific critiques of biomedical language ideologies, this capacity is at times explicitly recognized and embraced by biomedical practitioners themselves. The Conclusion thus underscores the critical role of language in medicine and the healing power of words.

# 1

# The Bottom of the Funnel

But the greatest thing by far is to have a command of
metaphor. This alone cannot be imparted by another; it is the
mark of genius, for to make good metaphors implies an eye
for resemblances.

—Aristotle, *Poetics*

If an electrical engineer could look at your neurological
wiring, he would see where the problem is.

—Dr. Novak

Suppose that a physician had decided that your pain was *all in your
head*. What, exactly, would that mean? When we label pain as "all in
your head," beyond merely specifying a physical location where pain is
thought to reside, we also draw on the head as a prevailing metaphor
for psychological phenomena. In the U.S. context, this metaphor is persuasive because it draws on widely held cultural models proposing that
illnesses are *either* mental *or* physical. Because the mind is the province
of the imagination, "all in your head" may also suggest that the pain is
made up or "unreal," the invention of a self-defeating mind, or, worse,
the fabrication of a malingerer. "All in your head" is thus a powerful
metaphor for illness because of the multiple meanings that it crystallizes
and collapses.

In this chapter, I examine the metaphors that clinicians use to explain
pain to adolescents and families. In her book *Illness as Metaphor*, the
literary critic Susan Sontag famously rejects the notion that serious illness
can be understood in terms of metaphor.[1] For Sontag, metaphors stigma-
tize cancer sufferers by cloaking a terrible disease in an aesthetic veil,
which, as it lends meaning, distorts. Sontag pleaded for society to strip

diseases of this symbolic content and understand them purely in terms of their biomedical meanings.[2] What Sontag's point misses, however, and what I seek to illustrate here, is that metaphors—aesthetic or otherwise—are endemic to biomedical practice itself and foundational to the ways in which practitioners understand and explain bodily processes.[3]

Here, I highlight in particular the pragmatic function that metaphors serve within clinical explanations. Drawing on interviews I conducted with clinicians on the West Clinic team, as well as other pediatric pain practitioners, I examine a set of metaphors used to present chronic pain as a problem of neural circuitry. Characterizing pain in this way addresses two persistent dilemmas that plague contemporary biomedical understandings of chronic pain: an ambivalent stance toward the role of individual psychology and the elusiveness of concrete causes. Metaphors for neural circuitry reconfigure the relationship between material explanations and biomedical legitimacy by replacing the fruitless search for mechanical dysfunction with a more diffuse model of nerve-signaling difficulties. Neural metaphors thus work to transform intractable pain from an abstract, senseless phenomenon to one that is meaningful, clear, and concrete. In doing so, they bolster the credibility of adolescent chronic pain sufferers, whose legitimacy and moral standing are routinely called into question when biomedical explanations fail.

**THE LONG ROAD THERE**

Before turning to these metaphors, it is important to say a few words about how families make their way to pediatric pain clinics. Chronic pain patients, including children and adolescents, are often referred to specialized treatment centers months or even years into their diagnostic journey, having seen multiple specialists and undergone scores of inconclusive tests, only to be told that there is nothing wrong, or, worse, that the pain is all in their heads. As Mark Siegel put it the first time we met: "In the past sixty-two weeks I've seen eleven doctors, nine of whom think I'm insane." Dr. Novak referred to the West Clinic as "the bottom of the funnel" because, as Nina Herrera, the clinical coordinator, explained it, "They've been to every pediatric subspecialty clinic; every test has been negative; everything's been cleared."

Most West Clinic patients found their way to the clinic after consulting at least three specialists—typically, gastroenterologists, neurologists, orthopedists, and rheumatologists. To families on a prolonged diagnostic odyssey, testing seems to offer a beacon of hope, a pathway out of uncertainty, yet in the case of chronic pain, it repeatedly fails to produce the desired result.[4] One mother referred to this thwarted quest as a journey through the "Bermuda Triangle" of pain, a metaphor that captures the aimlessness and sense of abandonment that many families experience as they search for help. Some disappear into the medical system, feeling rudderless and bewildered.

Mark Siegel's pathway to the West Clinic exemplifies the circuitous routes that many families take before finding their way to pediatric pain clinics. Mark lived in an affluent community with his mother, Julie, a pharmaceutical sales representative, his father Micah, who worked in marketing, and his younger brother, Noah. Mark's pain began after a boogie-boarding accident in August 2007, when he was thirteen, that cracked the growth plate in his left elbow. When the pain did not let up, Julie took Mark to an orthopedist, who diagnosed the fracture and put the arm in a cast. This was the third break to Mark's left arm: when he was six, he had fallen jumping off a jungle gym at school and broken the ulna and radius, and six months later, he had tripped and broken the same arm again. This history was significant because chronic regional pain syndrome (CRPS), the diagnosis that Mark eventually received, often occurs at the site of repeat injuries.

From the beginning of the latest injury, Mark was extremely uncomfortable. During the first nine weeks, the orthopedist changed the cast several times due to swelling, until he finally removed it for good. After that, Mark received physical therapy three times a week for ten weeks, but he remained highly sensitive to pain, and his physical therapist came to suspect that the arm had not entirely healed. However, when Mark returned to the orthopedist for further X-rays, no fractures were identified. The orthopedist encouraged the Siegels to "toughen up" on Mark, speculating that the pain would fade as he became more active. By February, his arm had still not improved, and he was complaining of pain more often. Julie brought him to two physiatrists, who recommended laser therapy, which Mark underwent twice weekly for five months to no avail.

Mark returned to his pediatrician, who referred him to a neurologist, Dr. Carmine, who finally diagnosed Mark with CRPS. Dr. Carmine ordered an MRI to make sure that Mark had not sustained any nerve damage and prescribed Neurontin, a drug initially developed to treat seizure disorders that is now widely used "off-label" to relieve neuropathic pain.[5] On Neurontin, Mark felt "loopy" but got no relief. Lyrica, another neuropathic pain agent originally developed for treatment of epilepsy, likewise offered no relief. Nearly a year after Mark's injury, he returned to Dr. Carmine for a third time. Now, because the medication trials had failed, she decided that he might be an appropriate candidate for a sympathetic nerve block.[6] The first nerve block was unsuccessful, and although the radiologist had suggested that it might require several attempts, Mark was reluctant to have a needle inserted into his neck again.

Meanwhile, during his recovery from the nerve block, Mark's blood pressure soared up to 168/82.[7] Julie brought him back to the pediatrician, who sent them to a cardiologist. The cardiologist ordered an EKG, which was normal, and an echocardiogram, which showed thickening on the left side of Mark's heart. The cardiologist then referred Mark to a nephrologist to rule out renal artery stenosis, a possible cause of high blood pressure in children.[8] Mark underwent several weeks of testing, but everything came back negative. However, because his blood pressure remained worrisomely high, he started taking a low dose of Enalapril, an ACE inhibitor, to lower his blood pressure. Julie and Mark were both convinced that his high blood pressure was related to his pain. Reflecting on this time, Mark said, "At the year mark it made me angry because my doctors have been idiots up to that point, not knowing what the heck is wrong with me. That a city with one million people doesn't have a doctor that can treat this is beyond me." Nevertheless, he believed that his best hope for recovery lay with medical doctors—he had tried alternative treatments such as acupuncture, herbs, and moxa with no success.[9]

When I met the Siegel family several days before Mark's first West Clinic appointment, they had begun to research pain programs and physicians in other parts of the country, afraid that they might have exhausted treatment options in their area. They told me about future plans to travel to a clinic in Northern California and to the Mayo Clinic in Minnesota, which they had put on hold when they found out about the West Clinic. In my experience, such travel was not unusual; several families traveled from out of state and stayed several weeks to have their child treated in the West Clinic. Julie reported that Mark was quite involved in the research process: "He gets on the computer himself, looking for pain specialists, and he's like, 'I gotta find someone that'll get me out of this pain.'"

In the face of Mark's increasing discouragement, Julie stressed the importance of his treatment. She said, "And he knows we keep trying and we keep calling doctors and we keep- you know, we're not giving up. And that's what we do, is we reassure him that we're not giving up. We're gonna try to get him—find him someone to get him the help he needs." For the Siegels, a big component of "not giving up" was financial: Julie reported that they had spent $4,300 between August and October alone. Yet Julie's investment was more than just monetary. She spent countless hours on the phone with physicians and pharmaceutical industry colleagues trying to get the best care for Mark. "I'm on the phone with doctors every day! Seeing what I can do. I'm on the Internet. I have not given up," she told me.

For Mark and his family, the West Clinic represented, if not the absolute "end of the road," certainly one of the last stops on a winding journey that included a narrowing range of possible destinations. However, while Dr. Novak's funnel metaphor might create the impression that all children and adolescents with chronic pain will eventually make it to a place like the West Clinic if they spin around long enough, this is not quite accurate. As with most health-care resources in the United States, access to tertiary care medical services such as specialized pediatric pain clinics is stratified according to families' insurance status and ability to pay. The story of fifteen-year-old Crystal Martinez, the first patient that I enrolled in my study, is quite telling in this regard. Although I recruited Crystal after her first appointment in the West Clinic was scheduled, she never actually became a clinic patient, because her Medi-Cal health insurance would not cover her treatment.[10]

Crystal's mother, Lucinda, a Guatemalan immigrant and single mother, was exceptionally devoted to providing her two U.S.-born daughters with the best available educational, extracurricular, and travel opportunities. The three lived in a two-bedroom apartment with Lucinda's sister and nephew in a part of town known for high crime rates, where the buildings were more weathered than in the Siegel family's community. A year and a half before we met, Crystal had come home from a school trip to Guatemala with body aches and a fever. When the fever spiked on the third day after her arrival back, Lucinda rushed her to the local children's hospital, where she was diagnosed with dengue fever and salmonella. After several months, Crystal had seen an infectious disease specialist and made two subsequent emergency room visits, but the body aches and abdominal pain remained. "They were not helping her," Lucinda recalled. "Whenever we go there it was the same thing. You know, Tylenol or [other] painkillers. I think they give her something really strong for the pain. But I don't want to give her that, because then she will get addicted to it."

At this point, Crystal's pediatrician referred her to a gastroenterologist in the same children's hospital, but the first available appointment was three months away. In the meantime, the family for whom Lucinda had worked since Crystal was six months old, as a nanny and then a housekeeper, suggested that Lucinda take Crystal to the emergency room at a different hospital across town and request that she see a gastroenterologist. Once there, Crystal was referred to a pediatric gastroenterologist, who eventually referred her to the West Clinic, located in the same hospital, when she ran out of treatment ideas.

The gastroenterologist prescribed Xifaxan, a short-course antibiotic that was not covered by Crystal's insurance, for which Lucinda paid $255 out of pocket. "We talked to [the gastroenterologist] about sending some forms but then in those days she went on vacation," Lucinda explained. "And the, uh, doctor that was . . . covering for her, ah, they didn't got the forms, and [when] they did got the forms, they send it to the insurance, they got lost. So whatever happens it just took a while. At the end, I never got any response from anybody, insurance or the doctor, so I just went in and paid for myself." I found Lucinda's experience particularly vexing because I had taken Xifaxan myself about eight months prior, and my own doctor, knowing that I was in graduate school, had told me that if my insurance would not pay for it, she would give me free samples. Lucinda was not offered these, and as a struggling single mother, the cost hit her hard.

Beyond the importance of financial resources, Lucinda and Crystal's experience also highlights the important role of what the sociologist Janet Shim calls *cultural health capital,* tacit or deliberate cognitive, behavioral, or sociocultural resources that predispose patients to optimal health-care encounters.[11] The suggestion by Lucinda's employers that she take Crystal to a different, more prominent hospital marked a critical turning point in Crystal's therapeutic trajectory. For working-class, non-native-English-speaking immigrants like Lucinda, the cultural health capital necessary to identify appropriate doctors and therapeutic pathways beyond ordinary pediatric care can be far out of reach. Prior to this point, Lucinda told me that, unaware of how to go about finding a suitable doctor in the United States, she had looked for a doctor for Crystal by dialing telephone numbers that she found in the Yellow Pages under "gastroenterologist."

Lucinda recalled this strategy as the most frustrating aspect of Crystal's medical journey:

> Find a doctor. Find a GI. That was so upsetting. I even went to the Yellow Pages and looked myself and tried to see a GI. And they said, "Sorry we can't take you because we only take from eighteen and up. Sorry we can't take

you." This is so frustrating. We find one that was gonna take us but it was, the appointment was for two months, and the visit is between 400 and up or 200 and up. Expensive. Which, I, like I said, you know, I don't mind the money you know, if it is helping her or is gonna help her, I will pay for the visit. 'Cause they say, "What plan do you have?" "Well I have this HMO, whatever." And they say, "Oh no, we don't take that." I say, you know, "It doesn't matter. I pay for the visit." And, it's start from—I think they said from 250 and up.

Despite Lucinda's resourcefulness, her willingness to incur substantial debts to secure medical care for her daughter, and her employers' willingness to help her financially, it was the relational currency of the latter's cultural health capital that proved instrumental in opening the door to better treatment for Crystal. Lucinda said of the wife, "She's the one who calls [the hospital], she's the one who calls here and helps me make phone calls. To help me get in anywhere."

Unfortunately, Lucinda learned just days before Crystal's first scheduled appointment in the West Clinic that her insurance would not, after all, cover the visit.[12] The West Clinic office visit would cost from $250 to $400, so they would need to postpone it. The West Clinic attempted to obtain authorization for Crystal's visit, but the insurance representative instructed Crystal see someone within the company's network first. When they updated me on this turn of events, Lucinda and the West Clinic receptionist formulated it somewhat differently. When I called Lucinda to check in with her, she told me that Crystal's appointment "had been canceled." I noticed this passive language choice because I had received an e-mail from the receptionist the day before indicating that the family "had decided to cancel." This subtle shift in agency highlights how, for many families faced with children's health-care needs, the notion of medical "choice" may be little more than illusion. If the choice really was Lucinda's, she was choosing between two undesirable options: keep the long-awaited appointment and take on a debt that she could ill afford, or forego it and attempt to find good care elsewhere.

Four months later, Crystal did obtain an appointment with a pain specialist at another pediatric pain clinic in the area, albeit one less renowned than the West Clinic. In this sense, Crystal's case was not a complete failure of pediatric pain treatment. Yet as I stayed in touch with Lucinda and continued to follow Crystal's therapeutic trajectory, it was clear to me that she received far less support and did not fare as well as many of the patients in my study, partially as a result of her family's limited financial means. Several months after Crystal's first pain clinic appointment, she suffered another treatment setback when the state determined that Lucinda no longer qualified for Medi-Cal and Crystal lost her insurance.

Crystal's experience demonstrates how, despite state and federal efforts that pay lip service to ensuring access to health care for all U.S. children, tertiary care pediatric services may nevertheless be construed as luxury goods that are not distributed equally. Patients like Mark were thus far more likely to make it through the West Clinic's doors than patients like Crystal. One reason for this differential access is the different levels of cultural health capital available to their families. Consider, for example, the ways in which the two families approached the task of identifying medical providers. While Julie queried her pharmaceutical industry colleagues, and Mark himself did Internet research, Lucinda adopted the less efficient strategy of looking in the Yellow Pages, until she received helpful assistance from her employer. These divergent pathways suggest that, if the West Clinic and others like it constitute "the bottom of the funnel," the funnel itself does not provide an opening that all families enter and pass through equally. As is typical in U.S. biomedicine, some never quite make it to the mouth of the funnel, while others remain permanently lodged in the neck, unable to get to the bottom.

## CLINICAL CHALLENGES AT THE BOTTOM OF THE FUNNEL

For families fortunate enough to secure a consultation in a pediatric pain clinic, the challenges are not yet over. Many adopt a cautious stance in their first visits, steeling themselves for yet another disappointment, however hopeful they might be. Families are especially likely to be guarded if they have been treated dismissively in the past. "If the family feels like they've been told that the pain condition has been all in their child's head," the psychologist Hillary Traynor told me, "they develop a real mistrust for working with care providers and even avoid that."[13] Dr. Joseph Stanley, the physician-director of a pediatric pain clinic in the midwestern United States, was more emphatic: "They're *always* skeptical and they're *always,* you know, 'We don't know what to expect. Every other doctor's told us that we're whacked in the head.' You know, or, 'People didn't believe us.' Or, 'No one's been able to help us.' They've all been through the medical wringer already, so they all come with baggage of one sort or another. And very few of them expect that we're gonna be able to help."

Referrals to numerous physician specialists, a seemingly endless stream of diagnostic testing, the tremendous burden of medical uncertainty, and insinuations that chronic pain is "all in your head" combine to put a great deal of pressure on pediatric pain clinicians to handle family inter-actions with great care and sensitivity. If pediatric pain clinics represent the bottom of the funnel, by the time families arrive, they have already been "through the medical wringer," as Dr. Stanley put it: spun around, siphoned through a narrowing range of treatment options, and spit out the bottom with nowhere else to go.

How do pediatric pain practitioners respond to this pressure? How do they explain chronic pain in such a way that patients feel validated? Metaphors provide a powerful resource for handling several interre-lated challenges that confront clinicians at "the bottom of the funnel." First, although the biopsychosocial model of pain eschews simplistic views of psychological causality, psychological factors remain impor-tant to the patient's experience and pain management possibilities. Yet questions about symptoms of anxiety and depression can easily send the message that clinicians conceptualize chronic pain as a psychological phenomenon, and thus not a *real* biomedical problem—particularly when families are predisposed, based on past experience, to view such questions suspiciously. The dilemma for pediatric pain clinicians, then, is how to convey to families that while they may inquire about a patient's emotions and mental state, which form an important part of the landscape of life with long-term pain, this does not (or does not necessarily) mean that they think that the pain is "all in your head." Dr. Novak addressed this directly with a favorite joke: "You may be crazy, but that has nothing to do with this."

A second challenge for pediatric pain clinicians is to manage expecta-tions for a concrete diagnosis. "They come to our pain program expect-ing, not necessarily a miracle, but they want a diagnosis—a lot of them want a diagnosis, a clear-cut diagnosis that can be treated," Nina Her-rera said. The assumption underlying repeated efforts at diagnostic test-ing is that the appropriate test—be it imaging, laboratory, or something else—can help to pinpoint a specific causal mechanism. The historian of medicine Charles Rosenberg has traced the emergence, over the course of the twentieth century, of a theory of disease specificity that conceptualizes diseases as concrete, isolatable entities that can exist, in his words, "outside the unique manifestations of illness in particular men and women."[14] It is precisely this understanding of disease that perpetuates the diagnostic odyssey: this logic suggests that there is something there to be diagnosed, and that eventually the correct test will identify it.

Chronic pain syndromes, however, often resist such specification. In addition to pain, the adolescents I met in the West Clinic frequently reported diffuse symptoms such as nausea, fatigue, insomnia, and even pseudo-seizures, as well as sensitivities to heat, cold, and sound. Consequently, their illnesses were not always clearly and indisputably linked to a specific organ or disease entity, but might be characterized instead with catch-all labels such as "central pain syndrome," a term used to express sensitization of the pain-signaling system, or generic categories such as myofascial or neuropathic pain.[15] Not surprisingly, this diagnostic fluidity sometimes left families unsatisfied. "They would be almost happier if you said, 'Your child has diabetes and needs daily insulin shots,'" said Deborah Vuolo, a psychologist working at a pediatric pain clinic in the northwestern United States. "Because it's concrete, and the problem with chronic pain is it's not concrete." Several patients and parents told me that it would almost be easier if the diagnosis had been cancer, because then there would be a clear treatment. What families feared most was, not a serious, devastating illness, but rather the complete absence of a concrete biomedical explanation—confirmation that the pain might really be "all in your head."

In what follows, I illustrate how the pervasive use of neurobiological metaphors in pediatric pain medicine works to address these interpersonal and explanatory challenges by finding an alternative vocabulary for pain that is "in the head," yet not psychological—in the sense of being "unreal" or made up. More specifically, I show how metaphors that conceptualize pain in terms of neural circuitry provide a compelling alternative to the doctrine of disease specificity by replacing the search for structural dysfunction in a particular organ with a more diffuse model of nerve-signaling difficulties. This model also helps to explain why other specialists have failed to grasp the problem: they tend to locate pain in a discrete body part, such as the stomach, head, or back, instead of in the nervous system. In laying out this alternative model of pain, pediatric pain clinicians provide a persuasive rationale for a novel mode of treatment based on "reprogramming" the neural circuitry. At the same time, neurobiological metaphors evoke tropes of techno-scientism and realism that are especially salient for middle-class Americans. In contemporary U.S. popular culture, neurobiology is widely and uncritically accepted as an agent of legitimacy that explains a wide range of symptoms and behaviors, and relieves individuals from responsibility and blame.[16] By developing elaborate metaphors to visualize and concretize a phenomenon that is notoriously difficult to represent, practitioners work to transform chronic pain from a perplexing set of loosely connected symptoms to a "real" illness condition.

It is important to keep in mind that neurobiological metaphors can serve to legitimize health-care providers as well as patients. At one pain convention that I attended, an audience member asked a well-known pediatric pain psychologist how he got families to accept his rehabilitation model of pediatric pain management. The psychologist responded that he always spends a lot of time explaining physiological pain mechanisms. "Your credibility goes up a lot if you do this, particularly if you emphasize the neural mechanisms," he explained. Striking here is the psychologist's suggestion that his own legitimacy, and not just the legitimacy of his patients' pain, was at stake in neurobiological explanations.

Metaphors are also common in pediatric pain medicine for another reason: they help translate complex concepts into terms that children and adolescents can more easily comprehend. Metaphors buttress clinical communication by capturing young patients' attention and helping them understand and remember complicated scientific ideas. Particularly in a domain such as pain medicine, in which there is so much complexity and uncertainty, metaphors draw on children's imaginative capacities to employ meaning creatively when it is otherwise underdetermined.[17] Explanatory metaphors for pain thus perform vital rhetorical work designed to counteract the evidentiary crises that surround pain.

## CLINICAL METAPHORS

When Dr. Novak describes her clinic as "the bottom of the funnel," she does not literally mean, of course, that the clinic is located at the bottom of a funnel. Instead, she suggests that the experience of pain treatment shares some of the funnel's properties and conventional meanings. The funnel metaphor not only suggests that patients and families are channeled along a constricting range of treatment options as the diagnostic odyssey progresses, but also highlights the lack of agency and control that they feel along this journey. Here, the metaphor works as a figure of speech that helps to provide conceptual clarity in virtue of its poetic properties.

Cognitive scientists, linguists, philosophers, and anthropologists have long observed, however, that metaphor is more than a poetic flourish; it is a critical mode of thought and action that pervades our everyday life.

In their classic text *Metaphors We Live By,* George Lakoff, a cognitive linguist, and Mark Johnson, a philosopher, argue that metaphor is a basic mechanism of the human mind that tacitly shapes how we think and act in ways that often go unnoticed.[18] At the most basic level, then, a metaphor is a form of representation that helps us to categorize the world around us.

Medical anthropologists have examined the role of metaphor in illness and healing from a number of different angles: by developing critical perspectives on the metaphorization of diseases;[19] by illustrating how bodily symptoms can express broader sociopolitical disorder;[20] and by identifying metaphors that serve as central organizing tropes in particular medical systems.[21] Anthropologists have devoted relatively less attention, however, to the functions of metaphor within clinical discourse. As linguistic forms, metaphors perform an important communicative function by encoding implicit assumptions about body and mind and lending concreteness to the inchoate, abstract, or elusive. In doing so, they produce "semantic movement" from abstract concepts to "more concrete, ostensive, and easily graspable" ones.[22] In clinical interactions, physicians, patients, and family members wield metaphors to help present a particular stance on a problem and persuade other parties of their perspective.[23] Such tactics are often successful because metaphors, beyond merely mapping analogical relations, transform the content of what they represent.[24] Furthermore, by endowing illness meanings with semantic flexibility, metaphors provide a convenient means of addressing the gap between available models of disease and treatment, on the one hand, and the experience of illness, in all its particularity, on the other.[25]

Given their utility in dealing with ambiguity and uncertainty, it is not surprising that metaphors pervade clinical discourse about pain. Metaphors are especially useful when ordinary language is stretched to capacity to perform its denotative function. This is why it might seem simpler to say that one's pain feels like sitting on a bed of nails rather than attempt to describe its qualities more objectively. Yet while many anthropologists have documented metaphors for pain in lay discourse,[26] few of these accounts have examined the metaphors that clinicians use as part of their explanatory armamentarium. It is to this task that I now turn.

### The Software Model

Early one September morning, I sat with Dr. Harvey Bergmann in his office before his staff meeting. Dr. Bergmann, the physician–director of a prominent pediatric pain program in the eastern United States, had invited me to sit in on the staff meeting and had agreed to be interviewed beforehand. The modest size and appearance of the cramped office, cluttered with piles of books and papers, reminded me of Dr. Novak's office, perhaps reflecting the humble status of pediatric pain in the medical hierarchy. Like many of the physicians I spoke with, Dr. Bergmann had trained in developmental pediatrics, a subspecialty devoted to caring for children with developmental, behavioral, and learning issues. He had also completed a year-long fellowship in psychosomatics, where he worked with a child psychiatrist to treat children with medical conditions and co-morbid psychological disorders. "This was a very long time ago," he said. In that era, he explained, there had been "very much a dichotomous kind of approach to many problems. It was either medical or psychological."

After accepting a faculty position and launching his career at an urban children's teaching hospital, Dr. Bergmann was often called in to assess the mental status and psychological functioning of patients with sickle cell disease. At the time, many clinicians believed that sickle-cell patients were all addicted to their pain medications, because they would ask for more drugs every few hours. "What really got me going with this was a thirteen, fourteen-year-old girl who was admitted to the hospital screaming in pain," he recalled. "And the question was: Was she addicted? Because she was requesting pain medications. And when I actually looked at her chart, she had had like five different pain medications, all of them inadequately dosed. She was watching the clock because she knew [that] every three or four hours she was entitled to new medication. Never treated adequately. So we changed her medication doses and she stopped complaining."

Nearly thirty years later, this incident still stuck with Dr. Bergmann. It had piqued his interest in pediatric pain and inspired the direction of his emerging research and clinical interests. In the intervening years, he developed an exemplary pediatric pain program, one of the first of its kind in the United States. More recently, he had shifted into the advocacy domain, working both locally and globally to, in his words, "create change in the culture of the institution." From Dr. Bergmann's perspective, it was not enough to rely on the "good graces" of individual physicians who understood the complexities of pain treatment; meaningful change had to come from the top down as well as the bottom up. Yet the cornerstone of his professional career remained his clinical practice, where he ran multidisciplinary inpatient and outpatient services for children and adolescents with chronic pain, as well as a consultation service for hospitalized patients with acute pain problems.

I was eager to ask Dr. Bergmann how he might explain pain to a new chronic pain patient, something I asked all the clinicians I spoke with. "So that's an interesting question, and I bet you'll hear amazing similarities, but everybody using different metaphors," he said. Dr. Bergmann motioned me toward his computer monitor, where slides for an upcoming grand rounds lecture on functional pain syndromes were already open on the screen. Flipping through the slides, he said:

> Because [other] people don't believe they're in pain, and they've been through lots of different people who disbelieve them, we tend to [tell them something like], "Your nerves have become hyper-aroused or overstimulated in some way, shape, or form." Rich Grostaurk talks about the habit of firing, the neuro-firing. Other people talk about the example people have heard of, phantom limb. But the model we use is that the nerves are overexcited for whatever reason. And we'll often use the software-hardware model. I don't know if you've heard [of] that model, too. So that's why everybody's looked inside of you, they haven't found anything wrong, it's because the software is the problem. And so what we want to do is figure out a way to reprogram that. And what makes the software—what got it going? Well, any number of things. A family history of this kind of problem might make you more vulnerable. We know that stress is responsible for all kinds of hormone production, and those stimulate the nerves. And yada, yada, yada, yada. And they're just firing, firing. So we get away from the psychosomatic. We get away from the dichotomous descriptions.

According to Dr. Bergmann, attributing chronic pain to neural arousal or hyperstimulation legitimizes it by establishing that it is caused by a concrete physiological problem. To illustrate this, Dr. Bergmann employed the central metaphor: "Chronic pain is malfunctioning software." This metaphor and its corollary—"Chronic pain is NOT malfunctioning hardware" in turn enable several key propositions that have important practical consequences for patients' understanding. First, other physicians have failed to correctly identify the pain because they are trained to address "hardware" problems—that is, problems with individual organs. Chronic pain results instead from problems with neural circuitry, which is here represented as "software." Consequently, other physicians (and their battery of diagnostic tests) have failed to explain the pain, not because it is "unreal," but rather because they lack the appropriate expertise. Second, the software metaphor provides a clear way of conceptualizing treatment as "reprograming." This model of treatment offers an optimistic prospect of recovery because software problems are generally easier to fix than hardware ones. Finally, the software metaphor exposes a range of potential causes for pain—from genetic predisposition to social stress—that provide viable alternatives to psychosomatic models.

I remarked that it must have been interesting for Dr. Bergmann to have seen the evolution of such explanatory models of pain, given his background in psychosomatics. He nodded in agreement. Had he been dissatisfied with the model available at the time, I wondered? "Well it made no sense," he said. "And also, the psychiatrists were lunatics. I hate to say it, but they were lunatics. You know, they would think that if you couldn't find a physical cause, there was a psych cause that was in there and we'll keep beating you. 'I think I see a little this or that,' you know, they'll make some crap up. You know, and they had this metaphor, you know, peeing. 'You're enuretic because you're peeing on your mother,' all this insane stuff. And I knew that they were nuts then. But there weren't good models then." Approaching the end of his slides, Dr. Bergmann summed up the appeal of his model: "So that's the model that we tend to use. And families respond to that very nicely because they don't feel blamed. They feel that, aha! This person understands the problem. . . . Most doctors say, 'Well I don't know what this is. But it's not this.' We say, 'We *know* what this is. We know what this is. We see this all the time, it looks differently in different kids, but we see this all of the time.' And that's giving people a reassurance that this is not a unique [phenomenon], that they're not the only one with this problem."

*"You've got pain!"*

My conversation with Dr. Bergmann was not the first time that I had heard a computer metaphor to describe chronic pain. Dr. Petrosian, Dr. Novak's junior colleague in the West Clinic, was especially fond of using the analogy of the Internet service provider AOL's well-known greeting: "You've got mail!" Invariably, when explaining pain to new patients, Dr. Petrosian would ask what e-mail server they used. If a patient said she used AOL, he might respond, "I use Gmail and Yahoo. You want to know why I don't use AOL? I check them when I need to. I don't like be told constantly, 'You've got mail!'" Here, Dr. Petrosian would mimic the grating voice that periodically notifies an AOL customer when a new message arrives in the inbox. He then would go on to explain how the neural networks that transmit pain signals start to develop patterns, firing irritating messages that say, in effect, "You've got pain!" over and over again, just like the AOL voice. "So we need to switch you to a new e-mail service provider," Dr. Petrosian would conclude, before laying out his treatment plan.[27] In this way, Dr. Petrosian's computer metaphors laid the groundwork for a particular kind of treatment: he often told patients that they needed to take their problem to the IT (information technology) people—meaning physical therapists, hypnotherapists, and psychologists.[28]

The AOL metaphor vividly depicts chronic pain as resulting from malfunctioning nerve-signaling circuits. When Dr. Novak spoke about neuropathic pain, she emphasized that it was a nerve-signaling rather than a nerve-damage problem. Thus, when a parent asked about surgical treatment options, she would often respond that you could cut the nerve, but the pain circuit would still remain in the brain, as in the phenomenon of phantom limb pain. As Meg Pratt, a West Clinic physical therapist, put it: "Amputate the foot, the person still has pain in their foot. It's not attached to their body anymore, so how can that be? How can they still have pain—feel pain—in their foot when their foot's no longer attached to their body? Because it's registered up in the brain." Dr. Novak also regularly told her patients that the nerve-signaling problem was the sort of problem that only an electrical engineer would be set up to fix. "That's why no one has found the cause," she once said. "It's not structural, not metabolic, not immunologic. The reason the tests did not turn up anything was that the diseases weren't there. And subspecialists don't get training in the neural networks of pain."

The importance of the distinction between nerve-signaling problems and nerve damage became clear to me one day that I observed a new patient's appointment with Dr. Petrosian. The patient, Phillip, was a ten-year-old boy who had developed CRPS in his right foot after a football-related injury. Dr. Petrosian explained that the pain was nerve-based, and as a result, the foot would not need to be put in a cast. Phillip looked at Dr. Petrosian with a puzzled expression on his face and asked, "So I broke my nerve?" Everyone in the examination room laughed, and Dr. Petrosian made a second attempt to explain the pain, this time using a football metaphor. Phillip had disowned his foot, Dr. Petrosian said, and he needed to retrain his brain to tell his foot what to do: "If you're tackling, you need to tell yourself to keep your feet moving. It's the same with this."

It is quite likely that Dr. Petrosian's second explanation was more successful than the first, because it drew upon a cultural schema that had personal resonance for Phillip.[29] Yet Phillip's confusion also highlights the dominant status of the body-as-machine metaphor in contemporary biomedicine. According to the anthropologist Cheryl Mattingly, this metaphor, which constructs the body as "potentially fixable," "operates virtually unnoticed in many clinical encounters."[30] It is only in moments when intersubjective understanding breaks down that the tacit assumptions underlying it are made explicit. In this case, Phillip's mistaken assumption that his nerve must be "broken" relates to a pervasive understanding of medical problems as occurring when the machine-body breaks, and of medical treatment as a matter of repairing a structural defect. In other words, the machine-body conventionally presupposes a mechanical fix.[31]

The computer-body suggests a very different kind of treatment, however. While a computer is also a machine, it is a specific kind of machine programmed to perform routinized functions. Rather than a mechanical repair, then, the computer metaphors described above conceptualize treatment as a recalibration of internal circuits and signals. Dr. Bergmann's software metaphor and Dr. Petrosian's clever deployment of AOL's signature line help to circumvent the doctrine of disease specificity by offering a different model of the body, in which pain is caused by underlying circuitry problems rather than "broken" parts.

In her work on views of immunity in American culture, the anthropologist Emily Martin tracks a parallel shift in metaphors for the body from the early twentieth-century view of the body as a fortress that must be protected from external penetration (e.g., by germs) to views popularized by the AIDS epidemic in the late 1980s that characterized it as a complex, flexible communicative system.[32] As Martin points out, the former model conceptualizes the body as a mechanical system composed of parts that can break down, whereas in the latter, body "parts" do not comprise the whole in a straightforward way. Rather, the body is constituted by a constant, fluctuating series of interactions that resist simple mechanical localization. Similar to the computer metaphors for pain, one of Martin's informants goes so far as to characterize the immune system as a "metabolic computer" that keeps the rest of the body in balance.[33]

One of the consequences of conceptualizing the body as a complex system is the paradox, as Martin puts it, "of feeling responsible for everything and powerless at the same time."[34] Like popular views of the immune system, the computer metaphors described above relay a paradoxical form of agency. As we will see further in the next chapter, a treatment approach based on "reprogramming" pain circuits, rather than structural repair, entails specific responsibilities for patients as well as their doctors. This differentiates pain management from the mechanical fixes sought in many areas of U.S. biomedicine, which tends to configure patients more passively. In this respect, computer metaphors for chronic pain also highlight the relational dimensions of pain treatment, demonstrating that therapeutic efficacy hinges on the patient's position within, and connectivity to, a particular social network.[35]

*Alarm Metaphors*

Thus far, I have suggested that metaphors for circuits and signals help to lay out a causal mechanism that attributes pain to a nerve-signaling problem and addresses why diagnostic testing typically fails to locate a cause. Yet another important function of metaphor, as I hinted at earlier, is its capacity to make abstract concepts concrete. Depicting chronic pain as the relentless voice saying, "You've got mail!" animates and concretizes a phenomenon that ordinarily resists such visualization. Another way of establishing that pain is real and not "all in your head" is thus to provide a set of metaphoric images that represent it as a material entity.

Consider the metaphor of pain as a burglar alarm that I heard from Dr. Sterling, the psychiatrist in the West Clinic, who explained:

> So here I am building a house and I take out my hammer, and I'm going to go to hammer a nail. And I miss the nail and I whack my finger. And I go, "Ouch, that hurts," right? But I've got to build a house, so, you know, I go back and I hit the nail and the next time I miss and I hit my finger again. And at some point, I don't actually have to hit my finger, but my brain says, Alan, you should probably put your finger away. And I can almost feel the pain, right. So there's a learning component to this. So that's the first thing I say. So there's pain information that goes from your finger, goes through the spinal column, and up to—there's a computer in the brain, which is monitoring everything we do, and memories and messages and all that stuff. And it says, uh, Alan move your finger, you're about to get whacked . . . So I think of it as an internal homeland security system. Like a burglar alarm.

In this account, Dr. Sterling uses metaphoric language to explain how the pain signaling system, when it becomes sensitized, may report pain that is not truly there. First, he provides an analogy for the conditioning associated with chronic pain: if you hit your finger with a hammer enough times, eventually the hammer alone can come to produce the pain response. He then offers two metaphors—an internal homeland security system and a burglar alarm—that bring these invisible neurosensory processes to life by anchoring abstract concepts in concrete visual images. The burglar alarm, a computerized monitoring system that warns of possible dangers, provides an apt conceptual metaphor for the nerve-signaling system, which monitors the body's sensory input. Like a burglar alarm, the primary function of the nerve-signaling system is to defend the body from harmful intruders, although "false alarms" are always possible.

Dr. Stanley described a similar situation using the metaphor of a smoke alarm. "There's supposed to be a set point, so your body knows when something's going wrong. And it's supposed to be like a smoke alarm," he explained. "And you know, much like your smoke alarm, you don't want it to go off all the time like it can when the battery's dead. And you don't want it to wait 'til your whole house burns down and your arm falls off to go off, either. You want there to be a set point so you know when your body is suffering from damage. But that set point can push out of balance." Much like the burglar alarm, the smoke-alarm metaphor suggests that chronic pain results from an overly sensitive set point that detects smoke when it is not really a danger. The concept of a "set point" concretizes the abstract notion of "pain as warning signal." The solution is to recalibrate the set point so that it detects pain at a more appropriate threshold. Dr. Stanley continued:

> You may still have a structural component. But that's not going to explain all of the pain that you're suffering from. There is this neuro-physiologic hypersensitivity piece on top of that. And that's really what in pain clinic we're focusing on treating. So we're not treating the underlying arthritis or treating the underlying structural defect in your shoulder. We're treating this neuro-physiologic hypersensitivity piece and you're gonna use a different way to get at that. So we're gonna use your body to get at it with the use of medication. We're gonna use your brain, the conscious part of your brain, to be able to be more in control of your nervous system as well and exert that control in a more constructive way.

The smoke-alarm metaphor thus paves the way for a particular kind of treatment that relies on the brain to control the nervous system. Although structural problems might also contribute to pain, they were not the focus of Dr. Stanley's treatment.

In this way, clinical metaphors enable specific possibilities for therapeutic action that map onto preexisting treatment ideologies. Because clinical explanations are necessarily "bound up with the practitioner's therapeutic imperative to act and his compelling need to rationalize his actions,"[36] causal metaphors for illness and disease can in some ways seem like post hoc justifications for a particular course of treatment.

This is not to say, however, that the practitioner's pragmatic motives here are purely self-interested. An important consequence of such justifications is the reassurance that intractable pain is treatable. For families who have been told that pain is "all in your head" and that nothing else can be done, the added value of an explanatory metaphor that concretizes the causes of pain and pathways for its treatment is the sense of relief that comes from feeling heard and understood.

In this respect, Chris Girard's recollection of his daughter's first appointment with Dr. Petrosian is instructive: "He nailed it, though, the first time we met you guys. He said several things that made sense which made it easier for us either, one, to understand, or two, explain it to people. And what she's going through now, you know, is the AOL account." His wife Shellie broke in, "You know, 'You've got mail'? That was big." Even though Dr. Petrosian had not been able to do very much for their daughter's debilitating pain symptoms, Chris and Shellie Girard recalled their introduction to him with obvious satisfaction, because he had explained her pain in a meaningful way. From this perspective, we might say that metaphors have an instrumental efficacy independent of therapeutic success.

### MEANING, CAUSE, AND THERAPEUTIC EFFICACY

However confident practitioners may sound when they explain chronic pain, the fact remains that the causes of chronic pain are often a mystery. As Hillary Traynor told me, "Sometimes we don't know exactly what causes chronic pain, but there can be illness or something physiologically going on that may cause kind of an overarousal of nerve pathways that may stay heightened after the illness is over, for reasons that we don't completely understand yet." Note that this response is full of mitigation and epistemic uncertainty: "we don't know *exactly*," "*may* cause," "*may* stay heightened," "don't *completely* understand." Such language underscores that chronic pain can be a baffling experience for patients and clinicians alike.

A central claim of this chapter has been that metaphors provide a rhetorical resource for clinicians to grapple with precisely this sort of causal ambiguity. Metaphors of circuits and signals are a powerful force in the West Clinic and pediatric pain medicine more generally. They help to address the uncertainties that pervade unexplained pain by providing a coherent causal framework that both materializes pain by representing it as a concrete entity and offers reassurance to patients and families that it is physiological and not psychological. Through concrete visualization practices, metaphors work to overcome the epistemological limits of the biomedical body, in which "to be 'real' is to 'show up' visually."[37] In other words, metaphors for the body can help to locate pain spatially when diagnostic technologies fall short. This rhetorical shift has moral implications, too. The ability to identify a concrete organic etiology—that is, to determine that pain is "real" as opposed to mental, emotional, and "all in your head"—helps to establish that a person is not crazy. Therefore, metaphors may help to validate accounts of suffering that have previously been met with suspicion.

Pediatric pain clinicians routinely turn to metaphors that substitute the metaphor of the body as a computer for the long-standing biomedical trope of the body as a machine. Depicting the body as an integrated network of signals and circuits enables clinicians to circumvent the doctrine of disease specificity and supplant the search for organ dysfunction with a model of nerve-signaling sensitivity. This also constructs bodily imaginaries that reflect broader cultural values surrounding labor and economy, as Emily Martin's work has also shown.[38] Computer metaphors that imagine one's body as hypersensitive suggest that, in our contemporary preoccupation with connectivity and flexibility, the pendulum may have swung too far, making us *too* responsive to changes in our environment. Yet far better to be hypersensitive, suggests this metaphor's implicit moral logic, than completely oblivious to potential environmental assaults, especially because in suggesting that one's nervous system is working too hard, this neural responsiveness evokes the cultural values of productivity and labor. Moreover, imagining the body as a complex system that can be recalibrated by IT experts draws on cultural ideals of techno-scientific enhancement and perfectibility.

The metaphors for chronic pain described here thus consolidate two intertwining temporal trajectories: a retrospective trajectory that explains pain in terms of its cause and a prospective trajectory that explains it in terms of its treatments. It is not simply the case, then, that clinicians first determine a cause and then settle on the appropriate treatment. Instead, metaphors for chronic pain reveal how the available treatment modalities prefigure certain causal explanations precisely because clinicians characterize pain in a way that renders it amenable to the therapeutic interventions that they can offer. For this reason, the meaning of pain is very much intertwined with therapeutic efficacy.[39]

Metaphors are intertwined with therapeutic efficacy in yet another way, however. In her ethnography of an inpatient pain-treatment center in Boston, Jean Jackson describes how metaphors for pain can be directly employed to great therapeutic effect.[40] In the treatment center Jackson studied, patients were encouraged to objectify pain by developing a visual image of it and then picture it entering and leaving the body. In imagining their pain as sea serpents, crabs, and medieval weapons, patients established a sense of control over pain: "The interaction between the pain image and the narrator frequently involved confrontation and struggle, requiring the pain sufferer to move from passivity to activity—even at times to risk danger and perhaps even more pain."[41] In this way, metaphors can become a powerful and productive therapeutic resource, illustrating that not just things like medicines but also words and images can have a healing effect on the body.

Although there is an abundant scholarly literature on metaphors for illness, mind, and body, underrepresented in this work are fine-grained accounts of what explanatory metaphors can accomplish in clinical discourse. As this chapter has shown, metaphors, as rhetorics of medicine, have the potential to reframe lay understandings of illness and harness positive, new, and valued meanings. Their persuasive power hinges on their semiotic properties as well as the social dynamics of the clinic. As I will explore further in the next chapter, patients buy into clinicians' metaphors in part because of physicians' authority.

If metaphors are a key element of clinical rhetoric, though, *how* do they persuade? Lakoff and Johnson distinguish between conventional metaphors that "structure the ordinary conceptual system of our culture" and a more imaginative variety "capable of giving us a new understanding of our experience."[42] That is, rather than merely describing our experience, they *transform* as they represent.

To illustrate this point, Lakoff and Johnson provide the example of a foreign university student they once taught who understood the American idiom "the solution to my problems" in strange yet evocative terms. The student had visualized this expression in terms of a chemical metaphor: a bubbling vat of liquid in which were suspended his "problems," in liquid or solid form. Depending on what catalyst one added to the solution, specific problems might dissolve or precipitate out. For Lakoff and Johnson, this metaphor offered a new, distinctive worldview, in which problems would never disappear entirely: "To live by the CHEMICAL metaphor would mean that your problems have a different kind of reality for you. A temporary solution would be an accomplishment rather than a failure. . . . The way you would understand your everyday life and the way you would act in it would be different if you lived by the CHEMICAL metaphor."[43]

The point for Lakoff and Johnson is not that words alone change our reality, but rather, that changes to our conceptual systems—to the *metaphors we live by*—can have this world-changing effect. For Chris Girard and his family, who had consulted seven specialists at multiple hospitals after a soccer injury left their daughter homebound with crushing leg pain, Dr. Petrosian's AOL metaphor facilitated a fresh perspective on pain that offered a renewed sense of hope for therapeutic possibilities. The Girard family's experience illustrates that changes to conceptual systems for making sense of pain constitute one of the most important therapeutic resources that families encounter at the bottom of the funnel, at this point in their diagnostic journey. Metaphors are thus critical clinical tools that perform essential rhetorical, interpretive, and therapeutic work. In this respect, clinical metaphors for pain offer a "synthesis of interpretation and creation"[44] that opens up vastly different perspectives onto reality. In the next chapter, I explore such world-changing metaphors in action by looking at a series of clinical interactions as they unfolded.

# The Smart Clinic

Models elicited by researchers from practitioners, in my
experience, tend to be considerably different from those
actually transmitted to patients or used to make day-to-day
clinical judgments.

—Arthur Kleinman, *Patients and Healers in the Context of Culture*

After eliciting his illness and treatment history, Dr. Novak
proposed to Jorge, "Let me see if I can guess your personality
and your mom and dad can confirm if I'm right." She said
that Jorge was probably very smart, sensitive, and eager to
please. Mr. and Mrs. Morales seemed to think that Dr.
Novak had hit the nail on the head with this description. Mr.
Morales even said that every year, Jorge's teacher always
says, "I wish I had thirty like him."

—author's field notes, October 13, 2008

Diagnosis remains a ritual of disclosure: a curtain is pulled
aside, and uncertainty is replaced—for better or worse—by a
structured narrative.

—Charles Rosenberg, *Our Present Complaint*

Zack Morgan had been screaming for days. Hobbling into the West
Clinic on crutches, he made his presence known by groaning and crying
out in pain every few minutes for the better part of an hour while waiting in an examination room for Dr. Novak to appear. When she finally
finished with the previous patient, Dr. Novak invited me to accompany
her to meet the family, suggesting that Zack, an eleven-year-old boy
who had been diagnosed with CRPS in his right foot, might be a good

patient for my research. Recognizing that this would be an interesting case to observe if not a particularly pleasant one, I warily agreed.

Zack was accompanied to the consultation by his parents, Jon and Sherri, and his twenty-one-year-old sister. Jon tried to maintain a sense of humor, joking about his willingness to leave Zack at the West Clinic and return for him the following week, but Sherri looked as if she had not slept in a week. Periodically throughout the visit, Zack would make loud noises that ranged from grunts to outright screams, and he often pulled his hair or knocked his head against his crutches, as if to distract himself from the pain by hurting himself further. Several times, he announced that he had an itch, and Jon stood up on cue to muffle the sound of his son's intense shrieks after Zack scratched his foot. Although disturbing to watch, this gesture was actually quite loving; Jon covered Zack in kisses as he bent over in agony. Remarkably, Dr. Novak carried on with the visit as if nothing were out of the ordinary, patiently collecting Zack's history in between shrieks, grunts, and cries. Later, she explained to the family that she was able to stay calm because she had seen enough similar cases to know that Zack was going to get better.

Zack described his pain as "burning, burning, burning, like someone is trying to rip my foot off." He was already on 1,500 mg per day of Neurontin, a high dose for someone his age and size, and 30 mg of Elavil, a tricyclic antidepressant commonly used off-label (i.e., for an indication, age group, or dosage for which it has not been officially approved) to treat chronic pain, in lower doses than used for depression. Sherri also indicated that she was giving Zack a quarter pill of Klonopin, an anxiolytic and anticonvulsant with sedative properties, twice a day to calm him down. The psychiatrist who had given Zack the prescription told the Morgans that this was all he could offer.

Zack had not been going to school, and this emerged during the visit as a significant site of tension, because he was anxious about what he was missing. Throughout the discussion with Dr. Novak, Zack fixated on three things: his desire to leave the clinic and go home immediately, his fear of shots, and his uncertain return to school. Sherri reported that Zack was often anxious when ill, and that she had considered seeking help for him to cope with anxiety even prior to the pain issue.

Aside from Zack's pronounced physical pain behavior, one of the most striking aspects of the consultation was a lengthy discussion of his character and its relationship to his pain. The following material is excerpted from the field notes I recorded at the end of the clinic day.

Dr. Novak asked the family to talk about what Zack had been like before the pain started. Sherri said that he was a fifth grader, a good student, and an amazing runner. Jon spoke about how Zack is a terrific artist and can see things in three dimensions, as well as a great guitar and Guitar Hero player. He loves science, "blowing things up," and puppies, in addition to watching *Family Guy* and *Seinfeld*. He is sensitive, polite, very respectful, and has lots of friends.

Jon also said that Zack is "very ethical." For example, he discourages Sherri from using her cell phone while driving, because it is against California state law. Sherri pointed out that Zack had protested when one of his sisters wanted to help the other with a paper for school because he thought such assistance was unethical. Jon shared an anecdote about how Zack was scheduled to have a cast removed from his foot on the same day that his class was visiting a pumpkin patch with their kindergarten buddies.[1] Zack refused to miss going to the pumpkin patch with his buddy because he thought it would be a very important memory for the younger boy and he did not want to deprive him of that.

Dr. Novak prefaced her explanation of Zack's symptoms by referring to kids who are smart, talented, creative, and sensitive. At this point, Jon interrupted to ask, "You mean the things that I told you before are relevant?" Dr. Novak nodded and explained that the neurobiology of kids with those characteristics is such that the brain makes lots of connections. She called this a neuromatrix and explained that it can lead to pain-signaling problems. Later on, Jon said that he was "blown away" by the conversation about Zack's sensitivity being relevant to the medical condition. (author's field notes, December 8, 2008)

### PERSONHOOD DIAGNOSTICS

Early on in my fieldwork, I realized that a large number of patients, including Zack Morgan, shared a particular constellation of characteristics that led Dr. Novak to refer to the West Clinic as the "smart clinic." They were gifted academically and usually talented in athletics or the arts as well. Often described as "straight-A kinds of kids," they tended to be achievement-oriented and driven (whether internally or by parental pressure) to succeed. They were also generally compassionate, sensitive, and empathic. Of course, this vision of what I call the "prototypical patient" is an ideal type: even those who did seem to fit the mold did not embody all of these characteristics. Nevertheless, the consensus among the pain team about the predominance of this type of patient was strong.

Over time, my clinical observations robustly supported this model. I met talented artists, gifted musicians, and accomplished dancers and athletes. One high-school student had secured a record deal to produce her first album. Another had been the only female permitted to play on an all-male baseball team. Yet another awoke before dawn everyday to attend an advanced calculus class that started at 6:15 A.M. Many seemed to be natural leaders in their schools and communities. They were, by all accounts, a rather exceptional group.

If I was fascinated by the question of why it might be that the "smart kids" would cluster in a pain clinic—a question that would likely require a different set of research methods for me to explore—I was all the more intrigued by the answer that Dr. Novak supplied to patients and families. As she explained it, it was this very constellation of features that primed them to develop chronic pain. There was something about "the neurobiology of being smart" that made them more susceptible to pain problems.[2]

In this chapter, I introduce the term *personhood diagnostics* to explore the ways in which Dr. Novak transformed the meaning of pain by embedding it in an explanatory framework that linked the neurobiology of pain to certain desirable attributes such as smartness, sensitivity, and creativity. By depicting patients in this positive light, Dr. Novak laid the groundwork from the first clinical meeting for a particular ethic of clinical care that privileged the patient's active responsibility for treatment. Within this narrative logic, diagnostic explanations reveal not only causal pathways, but also predictive claims about the likelihood of recovery, complicating prevailing psychosomatic accounts of pain.

Historically, psychosomatic disorders have been linked to a range of undesirable traits. Patients with conditions from neurasthenia to ulcerative colitis and even cancer have been described as overly sensitive, self-absorbed, and nervous.[3] Such characterizations of specific patient groups have flourished particularly when organic causes of disease cannot be identified. Although the links between illness conditions and personality types have sometimes been valorized,[4] these typifications have been framed overwhelmingly negatively. Chronic pain, in particular, has long been cast as a moral weakness. In the 1970s and 1980s, the psychological literature depicted "the pain patient" as a singular type: dependent, isolated, malingering, and self-defeating.[5]

Understanding people in terms of diagnostic categories raises key anthropological questions about how illness and subjectivity become intertwined over time and how institutional discourses mediate this process. Persons do not always fit neatly into prefabricated categories, and diagnosis risks reducing multidimensional individuals into flattened, prefigured types.[6] When identity and diagnosis are linguistically fused, as in the statement: "I *am* a schizophrenic," the distinction between "having" and "being" an illness is blurred.[7] In this formulation, identities are packaged in diagnostic labels: the patient becomes her illness.

Here, I use the term *personhood diagnostics* to highlight how diagnosis serves as a technique to categorize people, identities, and selves-in-the-making.[8] In anthropological scholarship, the term "person" designates a meaningful category in human social life that is tied to culturally and historically situated social roles, juridical rights, and moral responsibilities.[9] By foregrounding the moral and relational entailments of social (i.e., diagnostic) categories, I emphasize that therapeutic processes such as rehabilitation and treatment are imbued with institutional logics that demand personal responsibility for care and recovery.[10] The theatrical roots of the term *person* also underscore the fact that insofar as the prototypical patient was expected to embody a particular clinical and social role, Dr. Novak's explanatory framework mandated his or her performance in a largely pre-scripted therapeutic drama.[11] Therefore, I focus on the ways in which Dr. Novak's explanation of pain served to typecast patients into ready-made roles—for example, the "good kid" who was "Stanford-bound"—that held particular salience for adolescents and obligated culturally specific responses (e.g., to engage responsibly in self-care).

## EXPLANATION WITHIN THE CLINICAL ENCOUNTER

While the preceding chapter described clinicians' explanations of pain within interview accounts, my focus here is on how explanations take shape within the clinical encounter. In his foundational book, *Patients and Healers in the Context of Culture*, Arthur Kleinman emphasized the importance of examining professional explanatory models as they unfold in ongoing clinical interactions, arguing that it is insufficient for researchers to elicit professional explanatory models in interviews, because these models always lie at least partially outside of tacit awareness.[12] "Models elicited by researchers from practitioners," he wrote, "in my experience, tend to be considerably different from those actually transmitted to patients or used to make day-to-day clinical judgments."[13] In describing the models used in actual clinical practice, Kleinman distinguished between "clinical" and "scientific" explanatory models, asserting that for a clinician, "The choice of an [explanatory model] may be no more than ad hoc justification for use of one of a limited number of treatment alternatives or post hoc explanation of why the others were not tried."[14] From this perspective, clinical explanatory models are shaped less by scientific knowledge of a disease than they are by the practitioner's therapeutic objectives.

When faced with somatic complaints that elude established diagnostic categories and etiological knowledge, physicians may try to reassure patients or dismiss their concerns without explaining the cause of their symptoms satisfactorily. Psychological explanations can imply personal weakness and do not often lead to significant medical relief.[15] Yet simply acquiescing to lay understandings can risk undermining the patient's confidence in clinical authority.[16] Consequently, the cultural psychiatrist Laurence Kirmayer has contended that a balance between authority and invention is crucial to the success of the clinical encounter, to facilitate "enough closure or certainty to diminish the threat of the inchoate while preserving enough openness and ambiguity to allow for fresh improvisation."[17]

As Kirmayer's point suggests, representations of illness need not offer complete verisimilitude in order for them to be rhetorically effective. The anthropologist Claude Lévi-Strauss famously wrote of a shaman's apprentice, Quesalid, who discovered that that the efficacy of ritual healing depends on the sick person's belief in it: a shaman is only successful insofar as he can manipulate expectations of therapeutic relief. Quesalid's realization has significant implications for the anthropology of therapeutic processes. Cross-cultural studies have illustrated that one of the most effective aspects of symbolic healing is naming the patient's problem,[18] and that what the patient expects from treatments can have significant physiological effects.[19] Likewise, physicians draw on metaphors, images, and other rhetorical devices to clarify causal relations, assign meaning to symptoms, and rationalize a particular course of clinical action. In this sense, clinical explanations reflect ideological commitments and pragmatic circumstances as much as they do biomedical facts.

However, despite the importance of explanatory rhetoric in clinical interactions, anthropologists have paid relatively little attention to how it functions in biomedical settings. One reason for this omission is that explanatory models research has traditionally relied on interviews,[20] which fail to capture precisely the stories, images, and metaphors that clinicians use within ongoing clinical interactions. Furthermore, few studies in the literature on explanatory models have employed longitudinal methods to examine how patients' understandings of illness are transformed over time. By shifting the methodological focus to naturally recorded talk, I aim in this chapter to expand the analytic purchase of the explanatory models framework. Shared explanations do not emerge independently from the minds of patients and practitioners but are, rather, a product of recurring clinical interactions. In making this point, I engage with a long history of scholars who have argued that the joint production of meaning within talk-in-interaction is an important accomplishment of intersubjectivity.[21] Here, my focus on the real-time discursive construction of clinical explanations illuminates their pragmatic functions within clinical interaction.

In what follows, I examine how Dr. Novak's explanation of pain unfolds within real-time clinical practice. My pragmatic approach puts the analytic focus on the practical consequences of her explanation rather than its veracity. As the pragmatist philosopher William James has argued, "The truth of an idea is not a stagnant property inherent in it. Truth HAPPENS to an idea. It BECOMES true, is MADE true by events."[22] Focusing on a single case, I analyze the rhetorical processes through which chronic pain was causally linked to "the neurobiology of being smart," and, in turn, the patient was constituted as the type of adolescent who was capable of taking on an active role in the therapeutic process. I then return to Zack Morgan and his parents to explore the ambivalence that some families felt about this explanation of pain.

## THE SMART CLINIC

Michael Harris came to the West Clinic toward the end of a particularly tumultuous seventh grade year. The previous year, he had been bullied in his public middle school after sticking up for his best friend, whom other students had teased and called gay. When seventh grade began, this friend and several others transferred to a local private school and Michael was left alone to contend with the aggressors. Although Michael was almost thirteen years old, he looked closer to nine. His classmates taunted him about being short and having a high-pitched voice. "It was relentless," Michael told me in an interview shortly before his first clinic appointment. "One kid after the next."

In December, Michael developed severe abdominal pain, which his parents, and eventually he, came to associate with the stress of his school environment. By January, Michael had stopped attending school regularly, and later that spring he entered into a teleconferencing home-schooling program. Michael's pediatrician referred him to a gastroenterologist, who did a full workup of diagnostic tests, all of which came back normal. In the meantime, Michael became severely depressed, which both Michael and his parents attributed to his chronic pain, and Michael began seeing a psychologist and a psychiatrist. Michael's anger and frequent emotional outbursts soon began to overshadow family life. When Michael's pediatrician referred him to the West Clinic in May 2009, the Harrises were desperate for some relief.

As Michael saw it, the causal chain of his troubles ran from bullying to stomach pain to depression. That is, unlike many of the West Clinic families, Michael and his family subscribed to a model of psychological causality. Although they firmly believed that Michael's pain was real and not "all in his head," they did not think that it was rooted in an organic disease. Michael's mother, Kay, told me that when she scheduled Michael's appointment, she had said to the West Clinic receptionist, "You realize he has, like, no real *diagnosis,* right?" The receptionist had assured Kay that this was common in the West Clinic, and that Michael would fit right in. In some ways, then, the Harrises' understanding of Michael's pain made them more receptive than most families to the West Clinic's therapeutic model. However, as we will soon see, it also meant that Dr. Novak had to work to persuade Michael and his parents that the pain was caused by malfunctioning neural networks and was not a psychological failing.

Rob Harris, Michael's father, accompanied Michael to his first appointment. Although both of Michael's parents were very involved in his healthcare, Rob, a firefighter who worked continuous forty-eight-hour shifts separated by four days off, enjoyed a more flexible daytime schedule than his wife, Kay, who worked in the public school system. The first part of Michael's consultation consisted of a lengthy history-taking process, in which Dr. Novak invited Michael to tell his "story." Michael began by stating, "Well, it's functional abdominal pain, there's no terminal illness [*sic*] or cause for it. And we were thinking that it's caused by the bullying I had." As this comment suggests, Michael and his parents were well prepared to accept a psychosomatic explanation for his pain. Yet Dr. Novak responded by putting any causal attributions on hold: "Well, before we get to cause, let's focus on the experience of it."

As Michael spoke, Dr. Novak interjected with questions about his symptoms, treatment history, school, and social life, including how the bullying had started. Early in his account, it became apparent that Michael was academically gifted. He noted that his favorite subject was math (except for algebra), and complained about the incompetence of his classmates in the honors magnet program, indicting one child for his inability to do multiplication despite his advanced placement. "So you need the gifted-gifted class," Dr. Novak surmised. "Yeah," Michael agreed.

About an hour into the consultation, Dr. Novak diagnosed Michael with irritable bowel syndrome (IBS), a condition of unknown etiology affecting the activity of the large intestine, causing cramping, abdominal pain, bloating, gas, and constipation. Because there is no structural dysfunction associated with IBS, there are no specific diagnostic tests, and it is typically diagnosed only after more serious disorders have been ruled out.[23] In the excerpt below, Dr. Novak explains the diagnosis.[24]

EXAMPLE 1

Dr. Novak:  And what it is is, it's actually a real condition, it's not just cuz they can't find anything else

Rob:  Okay

Dr. Novak:  And what it is is, it's actually not in the intestinal tract, it's the nerve signaling bet[ween the brain and the gut.

Michael:                     [Yeah

Rob:  O[kay

Dr. Novak:    [Between the brain and the intestine. That's called a neuroenteric system. Nervous system. And what happens in IBS is the system becomes out of balance. The nerve-signaling system. So if we had an electrical engineer to look at the wiring we'd see where the problem is. So- we're not doing any tests. We don't need to.

Michael:  Not today

Dr. Novak:  No, not at all

In this initial assessment, Dr. Novak makes several important claims that lay the groundwork for her explanation of pain. The first concerns the ontological status of Michael's pain. Dr. Novak signals her intention to clarify the uncertain meaning of Michael's symptoms by twice repeating "and what it is is." She further reinforces the legitimacy of Michael's pain experience by assuring Michael that IBS is "actually a real condition." Here, "actually" functions as a contrastive epistemic device, asserting that IBS is real *despite* what people might otherwise presume. This claim is particularly important given the close temporal contiguity between the bullying and the onset of pain, which might seem to favor a psychological explanation.

Second, Dr. Novak specifies a spatial location: "it's actually not in the intestinal tract, it's the nerve signaling between the brain and the gut." With this contention, which has been widely cited in the scientific literature,[25] Dr. Novak helps to establish why the diagnostic tests thus far have remained inconclusive: they have been focused on the wrong anatomical system. Third, Dr. Novak provides a specific biological cause by stating: "what happens in IBS is the system becomes out of balance." The theoretical possibility that Michael's pain might be seen by an electrical engineer and confirmed through diagnostic imaging suggests that it is real, and rules out the need for further verification. Consequently, Dr. Novak declares, "We're not doing any tests. We don't need to." In the next excerpt, which occurred approximately two minutes later, Dr. Novak articulates the cornerstone of her explanation of pain: the connection between chronic pain and being smart.

EXAMPLE 2

Dr. Novak: And, um, ah, and so what happens is in really smart kids, you know, just like you learn things quickly, your brain makes connections quickly, you see things faster than other people may [or you get things faster

Michael: [Oh, your nervous system works faster

Dr. Novak: Your nervous system works faster. It gets it faster. But it also makes the pain signals get it faster.

Michael: Oh

Dr. Novak: So, u[m

Rob: [Ok[ay

Michael: [That's why reflexes aren't always a good thing

Dr. Novak: ((Laughs)) But it's gonna be good cuz it's gonna help you get out of it once you [know what to do

Michael: [O:::h

Dr. Novak: So this is the good- that's the good news. The bad news is you [more likely to get it but the good news

Michael: [Oh but if you get into something faster you get out of it faster

Dr. Novak: Exactly. Once you know what to do.

In the model presented above, Dr. Novak bolsters the status of IBS as a real condition by invoking "folk neurology."[26] Both smartness and chronic pain are attributed to "faster" neurobiological activity. Although, as Michael avers, high-speed neural signaling isn't "always a good thing," Dr. Novak transforms what could be seen as a neural glitch into a positive attribute by suggesting that it will also help him to overcome the pain more quickly. From this perspective, being a "smart kid" and a good student will also help Michael to be a good patient. Dr. Novak thus highlights the "good news," the positive side of an undesirable condition.

Michael, for his part, skillfully performs the role of the good patient/student. The frequency of overlapping speech demonstrates his attempts to participate actively in the discussion and anticipate where her explanation is headed. In doing so, he enacts the "smart kid" persona and gives evidentiary force to her explanatory logic. Dr. Novak's twice repeated phrase, "once you know what to do," prefigures the way that she will cast her role within Michael's ongoing treatment: as a supportive coach for his own self-care. Her primary task, from this perspective, is to provide him with the necessary skills to manage his own pain. About a minute later, Dr. Novak launches more specifically into the goals of treatment.

EXAMPLE 3

Dr. Novak: So the goal of treatment is two things. One to get that signaling system back in balance like it was before this all began.

Michael: [Mm hm

Dr. Novak: [And back to normal so you don't have to think about it or worry about it. And also to change the pattern of that, that memory map.

Michael: [Yeah

Dr. Novak: [Like to unlearn something or, or replace it with new learning actually

Michael: Almost like erasing words

Dr. Novak: Exactly. Gotta erase it and reprogram it.

Michael: Aright

Dr. Novak: Okay. So, um. And I'm gonna tell you what you need to do

Michael: [Oh right

Dr. Novak: [to help you do that. And because kids who are really smart can get it faster than kids who aren't

Michael: Mmm

Dr. Novak: You're gonna be able to learn this really fast

Michael: Aright

Dr. Novak: And change the program system

Michael: Okay

Dr. Novak: Okay. And make the pain go away.

Michael:      Aright

Dr. Novak:    And, and I'm gonna hang in there with you until it's gone

Michael:      Arighty

Dr. Novak:    And you don't have to think about it any[more

Michael:                              [Oh that'll be great

Dr. Novak again reiterates Michael's advantage: "kids who are really smart can get it faster than kids who aren't." By employing a treatment model based on learning, an implicit trope throughout this exchange, Dr. Novak draws on the specific strengths of the prototypical patient. Through her use of the second person future tense construction "you're gonna be able to," Dr. Novak assigns Michael three specific tasks that stress his active role in the recovery process: "to learn," to "change the program," and "make the pain go away." Accordingly, Dr. Novak provides not only an explanation of *why* Michael has developed chronic pain, but also a set of predictive claims about the outcome of his problem. In doing so, she pre-casts Michael as highly capable of carrying out a labor-intensive therapeutic protocol. This prospective orientation directs Michael's attention to a future without pain, beyond the confines of his present suffering. From this perspective, Dr. Novak's explanation offers more than a causal account: Michael will be able to get *out of* pain for the very same reasons that he has gotten into it. Once again, Michael performs the role of the good, compliant patient by responding to her account with positive continuers ("Yeah"; "Aright"; "Okay") and endorsing her overall plan ("that'll be great").

In contrast to Michael's active stance and therapeutic responsibilities, Dr. Novak defines her own role as to provide a supportive, coaching role: "to hang in there with you until it's gone." In doing so, she delineates an ethic of care whereby Michael has both the capacity and the responsibility to take center stage in his own treatment. Although this emphasis on self-care might appear to suggest the deflection of clinical responsibility, the crucial affective value of Dr. Novak's support should not be underestimated. Her reassurance that she will stay with her patients until the pain subsides addresses the fears of abandonment that many chronic pain patients develop over time, when they are passed off to yet another clinician because the first one thinks all her options have been exhausted. In this sense, what might seem to be a passive stance toward treatment might also be described as an active affective engagement. Dr. Novak's diagnostic schema thus reveals moral sensibilities about how persons are obligated to participate in medical care.

## PHARMACEUTICAL IDEOLOGIES IN THE WEST CLINIC

Before examining how Dr. Novak articulated Michael's treatment plan, it will be helpful to have some background information on the West Clinic's views on pharmaceutical treatment. Although the West Clinic's therapeutic approach assigned patients an active role in treatment, pharmaceuticals were still a critical component of treatment in the clinic. Dr. Sterling, the clinic's psychiatrist, joined the pain team around the same time that I began my fieldwork, and several clinicians were quite vocal about the value of his pharmacological knowledge, noting that he filled an important niche on the team that had remained unoccupied since the previous psychiatrist had left the clinic several years prior. The clinic's supportive stance toward pharmaceuticals was informed by the recognition that children's pain is often undertreated and an ethical commitment to redress this undertreatment. Yet it was also accompanied by several caveats, as we will soon see.

In general, the physicians tried to avoid opioids, though several patients did take drugs such as Oxycodone and Vicodin. While mounting anxieties surrounding an emerging "epidemic" of opioid abuse have contributed to greater restraint in prescribing these medications for adults,[27] for pediatric patients, clinical concern focused especially on the dangers of introducing potentially addictive medications at such an early point in their lives. As one medical student who rotated through the West Clinic explained to me, "Maybe you can do that in an adult population, it's a little easier with adults, but you still don't want to give a little kid like tons of Vicodin and tons of, you know, pain meds." When I asked why not, she replied, "Because, I think, of the risk of addiction. You know, you just don't know, like, opiates, you're gonna develop tolerance and you don't want them to down the line develop tolerance and not be able to use the pain meds if they're really necessary."

Opioid replacement therapy was a standard alternative to opioid analgesics, if not a particularly common one. Replacement therapies, such as methadone and the newer drug Suboxone,[28] are employed both to treat opioid addiction and to treat chronic pain, objectives that overlap in complicated ways. Championed for their "ceiling effect," which means that their effects are not intensified at higher doses once they reach a certain plateau, they enable patients to reduce the use of opioids without experiencing withdrawal symptoms. One of the particular assets that Dr. Sterling offered the West Clinic was that he had undergone the legally mandated training necessary to prescribe Suboxone in the United States.[29]

If opioids and replacement therapies constituted the more extreme end of the pharmaceutical spectrum, more common choices included medications such as Neurontin and Lyrica, both initially designed to treat seizure disorders. A variety of antidepressants were also quite commonly used, particularly selective serotonin reuptake inhibitors (SSRIs) such as Lexapro and Celexa, which were the preferred first-line pharmaceutical treatment for patients with symptoms of anxiety. Despite the frequency of co-morbid anxiety and depression in this population, use of these drugs was typically rhetorically framed for patients and families vis-à-vis the critical role of serotonin in responding to pain; sometimes the fact that they were antidepressants was not mentioned at all. Elavil was also prescribed, commonly at very low doses, especially for abdominal pain and headaches. Occasionally, stronger anxiolytics such as Xanax and Klonopin or even antipsychotics were prescribed on a short-term basis. For example, at Zack Morgan's first visit to the West Clinic, Dr. Novak gave him a small dose of Seroquel, an antipsychotic approved for the treatment of bipolar disorder and schizophrenia.

As may be clear from this discussion, pediatric pain medicine relies heavily on off-label use of pharmaceutical treatments. From an anthropological perspective, this may appear to be evidence of pharmaceutical company overreach,[30] particularly in light of well-publicized controversies such as the one surrounding Pfizer's allegedly fraudulent marketing of Neurontin and Lyrica, for which it has paid several hundred million dollars in settlements.[31] Yet for several reasons, I am wary of falling too easily into a critical social-science stance in interpreting what some readers may see as an extraordinary use of off-label medication. First, due to ethical concerns about enrolling children in research, fewer pharmaceutical studies are done with children and adolescents, making it harder to obtain approval for this population from the Food and Drug Administration (FDA). Consequently, much prescribing for children and adolescents falls into the off-label category. Secondly, many drugs that are used off-label to treat chronic pain are safer and less addictive than their FDA-approved counterparts (such as opioid analgesics), particularly for use in children and adolescents. And finally, in my experience, drugs such as Neurontin frequently (though not always) helped patients tremendously.

Nevertheless, despite the use of a wide range of pharmaceutical agents, the West Clinic team was firmly, and unilaterally, committed to a clinical ideology which held that medication alone was insufficient for treating chronic pain. As Dr. Novak reportedly told one parent, "We can pour a whole pharmacy into your daughter, but unless you guys work on the family issues, it's not going to matter." More specifically, medication was seen to offer the immediate relief necessary for patients to engage in longer-term therapies. Arlene Weiss, a psychologist on the team, explained, "I think sometimes if somebody is anxious or very depressed, it's very hard to commit or be motivated if you just feel out of control. Or you feel sort of oppressed by a depression. So I think until you've treated some of the symptoms, it's hard to get somebody motivated to start working and using some of the other approaches." However, while medication might jump-start the therapeutic process, the prevailing clinical wisdom held that patients were unlikely to experience lasting relief without a personal investment in additional pain management strategies. As Rebecca Hunter, the family and child therapist, put it, "I often talk to them about, you know, that I don't trust as much when it's an overnight miracle kind of cure because then I feel that they haven't built up the skills or, um, the ability to control it in the future if it happens."

Some patients struggled to balance such motivational goals with the sedating properties of pain medications. Seventeen-year-old Brandon Rothschild observed that methadone "drugged" him enough to enable him to visit to a university-based physician who practiced traditional Chinese medicine—who urged him to discontinue the methadone. In this case, then, the short-term course of medication, which his mother dubbed a "methadone vacation," served its higher purpose. However, the opioids that were meant to give twelve-year-old Jorge Morales enough relief to engage in physical therapy made him so tired that he never wanted to get up off the couch, let alone do his exercises. It was therefore sometimes difficult for families to know whether they were trading one set of problems for another.

Clinical reservations about pharmaceutical treatment were informed by a number of additional factors. Most West Clinic patients had already tried a long list of medications before arriving in the clinic, so the prescribing physicians were often limited in the number of new drugs they could try. Moreover, pediatric pain patients tend to react strongly to small changes in medication, which the clinicians explained in terms of the sensitivity of their nervous systems. "We use micro, almost homeopathic doses of medicines, 'cause the brains of these kids are so sensitive," Dr. Sterling told me. "What I've learned is, you know, you have to divide everything by ten when you start prescribing [for these patients]. . . so I've really had to restructure my thinking." A range of undesirable side effects, from hallucinations to weight gain to acne, went hand in hand with this sensitivity, sometimes making it difficult for physicians to find a suitable medication.

Finally, and perhaps most important, West Clinic families were sometimes reluctant to have their children take certain medications. Sometimes there were addictions in the family, and several patients had a history of addiction themselves. Others were familiar with the substance-abuse problems of friends or acquaintances and were therefore wary of taking these medications.[32] On still other occasions this resistance appeared to result from the prominent role of psychotropic drugs in U.S. culture. Nina Herrera, the clinical coordinator, noted that she occasionally entertained questions from parents about Prozac because of its name recognition, following its popularization in the United States during the 1990s. "Our typical answer, which is usually the case, is that we're not treating depression," she explained. "We're not using the medication in the dosage required to treat depression. It's treating the pain." To mitigate this stigma, Dr. Novak typically framed pharmaceutical treatment with precisely the same metaphors that she used to explain other therapeutic mechanisms, suggesting that it worked to calm down the nervous system or reprogram the pain-signaling network.

## SHIFTING PARADIGMS

It is against this pharmaceutical backdrop that Dr. Novak's explanatory rhetoric of pain treatment must be read. After hearing her use language similar to that employed with Michael Harris in more than a dozen clinic intake appointments, it was clear to me that her diagnostic performance was, at least to a certain extent, scripted. Yet it was not until I interviewed her toward the end of my study that she articulated an explicit rationale for explaining chronic pain and its treatment in this manner. On a sunny afternoon in early July, just as summer seemed on the cusp of arriving, I sat with Dr. Novak in the shade of an umbrella in her backyard. When I mentioned that I had noticed that she seemed to have a standard way of explaining pain to her patients, she told me: "Part of the goal of the first interview, besides allowing patients to tell their story, and listening, is also to change their paradigm about pain. And I sort of feel like, if I can't really do it and help them change it in that first meeting it's gonna be—I mean, there's times when they sorta get it, and then you have to remind them again later, but if they just don't buy it right up front, my experience is they probably never will."

As Dr. Novak saw it, the first clinic appointment presented an exclusive opportunity to shift the patient's orientation from an exclusive focus on curing pain with the right medication to longer-range strategies of pain management. She elaborated: "It's sort of trying to set the stage for why the goal of treatment isn't: you have pain, take this pill, and you'll be better. But. . . how emotions and thinking . . . all of these things are important and how they all relate to pain, and unlike acute pain, it's not just get rid of the pain and then they can go to school. It's: you have to go to school, learn to cope with the pain, and then, you know, et cetera. So it's—I just feel like that's an important part of helping them become motivated to engage in the various therapies."

The shift to a biopsychosocial paradigm of pain management entailed certain obligations for patients: to attend school despite suffering, to learn to cope with the pain, and to commit to various therapies. In turn, these obligations entailed responsibilities for parents—such as paying for multiple therapies and driving children to appointments—and required that Dr. Novak persuade parents as well as patients of the importance of the clinic's resource-intensive treatment approach. From this perspective, her explanatory framework was specifically designed to provide a foundation for a particular paradigm of pain treatment—and crucially, one that stood to fly in the face of parental desires for a pharmaceutical solution. In fact, Dr. Novak worked to render pharmaceutical solutions less desirable through the image of the "magic pill," a recurrent trope throughout our discussion. By situating purely biomedical treatment in the realm of fantasy, the "magic pill" performed a rhetorical inversion: it symbolically transformed a biological substance into an imaginary entity.

Intrigued by Dr. Novak's frank disclosure about her explanatory framework and its pragmatic function, I pressed her further to describe how she had come up with it. She continued:

> I think pictorially . . . maybe from all of my early hypnotherapy work,[33] I use stories and metaphor as often as I can. And so, that's why, you know, if you talk about stress, anxiety, how does being smart have a role in pain? So I try to talk about it as, well, it's a risk factor, but here's the good news. So, you know, [I use] the idea [that] if you learn quickly, your brain makes connections quickly. . . . That's how pain connections get set up quickly. The good thing is, once you know what to do, you make the connections not to do that [be in pain] quickly.

As Dr. Novak insinuates here, using explanatory devices such as pictures, stories, and metaphors works to concretize a phenomenon that is notoriously difficult to represent. Evelyn Fox Keller suggests that scientific models may "make productive use of the imprecision of metaphor and other linguistic tropes" when explanations prove elusive.[34] Drawing on work in physics and developmental biology, she argues that many scientific models are not grounded in empirical observation, but instead emerge from a process she calls "theoretical imagining." While these models may idealize and simplify scientific truths, they also contribute to conceptual clarity and enable the development of new knowledge. Similarly, images like Dr. Novak's electrical engineer in Example 1 above—"So if we had an electrical engineer to look at the wiring we'd see where the problem is"—might best be viewed as imaginative constructions designed to concretize and clarify the puzzling aspects of pain.

Dr. Novak's use of neurobiological tropes can also be understood as part of an effort to legitimize her patients' suffering. However, despite the allure of neurobiological explanations, there is a central tension between Dr. Novak's diagnostic logic and her therapeutic plan: while she carefully articulated Michael's pain as a biological problem, her therapeutic approach rejects the biomedical paradigm's purely technical fix. In framing his IBS as a "real" biological problem, she is aware that it is rarely effectively treated with biomedicine alone.[35] In order to justify a therapeutic paradigm in which patients use multiple therapeutic modalities to take control of their own healing, Dr. Novak must convey that her recommended course is just as legitimate (i.e., biological) as the pharmaceutical option. We will see how she does this next.

### SCIENTIZING TREATMENT

Returning to the clinical scene where we left Michael, Dr. Novak had just identified the goals of treatment: to *erase* and *reprogram* his neural signaling. Because Michael was already seeing a psychiatrist, who had recently started him on Celexa, Dr. Novak suggested that she talk to the psychiatrist about possible medications, explaining that she wanted all of the medication to be coordinated through one physician.[36] Celexa had been a good choice for Michael, she said, because it helped relieve stomach pain as well as depression. She then raised the possibility of starting Michael on an additional, temporary medication, "to make things move a little faster."

EXAMPLE 4

Dr. Novak: There are two options. Two different pathways and just so you know what I'm gonna talk with her about. And then we'll talk about nonmedication things. Um, one is (.) Risperidone,[37] which is a- and it would be in a teeny teeny dose just at night, just to quiet down that um that set-off valve

Rob: K[ay

Michael: [A:w

Dr. Novak: Just so that um things- or it gives a little extra buffer for things getting inside

Rob: Okay

Dr. Novak: So you know, that catastrophizing

Rob: [Sure

Dr. Novak: [that worrying, that then makes the pain, [you know.

Michael: [And what about the- I'm more worried about the depression than the pain.

Dr. Novak: Um, they're all, [this

Michael: [Oh

Dr. Novak: They're all connected

Michael: Alright

Dr. Novak: I mean, we're talking about all three. Depression, worrying, and ah, [the pain

Michael: [pain

Dr. Novak: Cuz they're all very much connected

Michael: Alright

Dr. Novak: A lot of the same neurotransmitters and neural signals. And so the question about that versus being on um very low dose what's called a benzodiazepine like Klonopin

Rob: Mm hm

Dr. Novak: Just to get at worrying catastrophization. Because

Rob: [Okay

Dr. Novak: [they're so linked together that they're different pathways of getting at it

Michael's question about Dr. Novak's apparent targeting of pain instead of depression offers an important window onto his compelling concerns, since this is the first time in the visit that he has expressed any sort of resistance to Dr. Novak's explanation and treatment plan.

Dr. Novak, in turn, models a particular relationship between pain, anxiety, and depression that views these symptoms as interconnected at the level of cause ("a lot of the same neurotransmitters and neural signals") as well as the target of treatment. As Dr. Novak presents it, quieting down "that set-off valve" would both dampen Michael's problematic emotions and minimize his pain.

After this brief discussion of pharmaceutical options, Dr. Novak went on to describe two "nonmedication" therapies that she thought would be useful: hypnotherapy and acupuncture. In the following account, we see how Dr. Novak begins to construct an account of hypnotherapy that upholds Michael's responsibility for his treatment while simultaneously grounding its therapeutic efficacy in scientific principles.

EXAMPLE 5

Dr. Novak: One is to use your smarts to start changing that patterning in your brain. So to start turning off both the depression and the- and I'll tell you how to do it. Um, the depression and the pain signal- member I said how that

Michael: [that it's a pattern

Dr. Novak: [a lot of the- that pattern is there. Just like you learn how to ride a bike and then you just- it's there already but you don't even think about riding a bike

Michael: (xxx)

Dr. Novak: You already know how to ride. Well your brain already knows how to have stomach pain and it's going whether you want it or not so we need to unlearn that, and change that pattern

Michael: Mm hm

Dr. Novak: So there's, um, something called uh using imagery, using the part of your brain and strengthening the part of your brain that thinks with pictures

Michael: Mm hm

As in the previous example, treatment is presented as recalibrating the pain system, whether by tweaking the "set-off valve" through medication or "changing that patterning in your brain." These explanatory models of treatment depict pharmaceuticals and hypnotherapy as operating in similar ways, putting them on an equal footing with respect to therapeutic efficacy. Furthermore, learning to ride a bicycle here serves as a metaphor for the habituation associated with chronic pain. By framing pain as something that develops outside of personal agency, "whether you want it or not," Dr. Novak creates a subtle distinction between actions of the person and actions of the brain. Moreover, by imputing agency to the brain and endowing it with human capabilities, such as "knowing," Dr. Novak also contributes to the "personification of the brain."[38] Insofar as such splitting between person and brain mitigates personal responsibility for illness, it serves an important rhetorical function: it diminishes the possibility that Michael might be blamed for his pain. Once again, Dr. Novak reiterates that Michael's intellectual capacity will be crucial to his ability to overcome these faulty neural networks by "strengthening" the brain. By articulating her treatment plan within this neuroscientific register, Dr. Novak works—in her words—to "biologicalize" hypnotherapy. This language helps to create a sense of biomedical legitimacy, which might otherwise be lost in a psychosomatic account.

In the following example, Dr. Novak works more specifically to construct hypnotherapy as a brain-based therapy. After asking Michael to imagine several characters from his favorite television show to demonstrate his capacity to "think in pictures," Dr. Novak continues with her explanation.

EXAMPLE 6

Dr. Novak: So it's the part that's in your head, that part of your brain, we know can start overwriting, and it's like, it's like erasing the pattern

Michael: [How would that happen

Dr. Novak: [and creating a new pattern through using imagery

Michael: But-

Dr. Novak: with something called hypnotherapy

Michael: Oh, I like hypnotherapy=

Dr. Novak: =And uh Charlotte Lefevre who's part of our program is- she works out of her home which is in [*name of town*] so you just park right outside and go in, makes it easy. Um, and she is a master at helping you learn to start erasing that and replacing

Michael: [I'm-

Dr. Novak: [that. And it sounds weird but you will [have fun

Michael: [I'm skeptical so

Dr. Novak: Oh of [course

Michael: [very skeptical

Dr. Novak: Of course. And I expect you to be skeptical

Michael: I'm skeptical about almost everything, so

Dr. Novak:   Well that's fine, and I'm used to that

Michael:     Skep-

Rob:         ((Laughs))

Dr. Novak:   You know, think of it as, as a- being um a scientist

Here, Dr. Novak relies on computer lingo and scientific references to assert Michael's ability, through imagery, to create new patterns in his brain by "overwriting" preexisting patterns. By characterizing the therapeutic process with an emphasis on learning, Dr. Novak depicts Michael as an active agent of his own recovery who needs only the guidance of a supportive "master." Dr. Novak does not demand that Michael accept her ideology unquestioningly. She acknowledges that it "sounds weird," and when Michael expresses reservations, she validates his cynical stance and concedes that she expects him to be skeptical. Yet by encouraging him to approach this novel situation as a scientist and permitting him to reserve judgment until he tests it himself, Dr. Novak supplants her own authority to scientific observation. In doing so, she creates a sanctioned space for doubt and empirical verification, both important components of scientific practice.

At the same time, casting Michael's treatment role as that of a scientist makes creative use of his "smart kid" persona. Michael likewise portrays himself as an active, engaged patient by asking questions ("How would that happen?") and expressing polite yet critical feedback rather than accepting her explanation passively. In doing so, he actively inhabits the particular subject position that Dr. Novak has carved out for him. This excerpt thus illustrates how Dr. Novak deftly deploys personhood diagnostics in the service of treatment uptake.

. . .

Michael seemed quite receptive to Dr. Novak's explanatory framework and therapeutic approach from the start, but an exchange that occurred during a clinical consultation two months later demonstrated the extent to which he had incorporated the treatment model into his own understanding of pain. In the following example, drawn from Michael's third appointment in July 2009, Dr. Novak seizes an opportunity to attribute Michael's improvement to his hypnotherapy work with Charlotte, whom he had visited weekly following his first appointment. As we enter the scene, Michael's mother Kay has just prompted Michael to give Dr. Novak an update about his akathisia, a side effect of the Celexa that Michael described as an unpleasant, skin-crawling sensation.

EXAMPLE 7

Kay:        How's your akathisia?

Michael:    Akathisias are fine. They're minor. As they were. They don't happen- they happen every day but they're like five ten minutes at a time. Small. Like, I can walk right through them, so.

Dr. Novak: So manageable?

Michael:    Yeah. But then again I have learned to experience pain much much better than I used to. Cuz I mean whenev- like whenever something hurts I'm like, like stubbed my toe this morning, like (.) that's not usually what happens.

Dr. Novak: ((Laughs))

Michael:    So I go, ow, it's gone. I'm like ((looking up at ceiling))

Dr. Novak: So wow, it sounds like your work with Char[lotte

Michael:                                              [Ye:s

Dr. Novak: is really chan[ging

Michael:                  [It is

Dr. Novak: all that cir[cuitry

Michael:                [It is

Dr. Novak: That's great

Michael:    It is, it is

Here, Michael happily describes how a stubbed toe no longer provoked a prolonged pain response, as it might have in the past; instead, the pain subsided almost immediately. Without skipping a beat, Dr. Novak attributes this transformation to Michael's work with Charlotte, thereby reinscribing therapeutic efficacy within a specific local understanding of the neurobiological mechanisms of pain. By suggesting that Michael's pain response has improved because he has successfully changed his neural circuitry, Dr. Novak frames Michael as the consummate patient, an active agent of his own recovery.

Michael's own behavior throughout this interaction provides some indication that he has accepted responsibility for his treatment and recovery. Although his affect starts out somewhat flat at the beginning of the interaction, because he had been arguing with his mother, he becomes visibly more excited as Dr. Novak gives her account, turning his gaze to her, nodding his head in agreement, and smiling. At the same time, "it is" directly confirms Dr. Novak's suggestion while also expressing ownership, providing stronger agreement than a mere "Yes," while his prosody—the rhythm and intonation of his speech—also quickens, suggesting excitement. Michael's uptake thus demonstrates the convergence of practitioner and patient on a shared explanation of pain.

Although a more cynical reading of this scene might suggest that Michael was merely eager to *appear* as a good patient, Michael and his parents told me that Michael did in fact attribute a large degree of his improvement to his work with Charlotte. Their explanatory convergence was underscored by the gratitude that Kay and Rob expressed for Dr. Novak's explanatory account during Michael's fourth clinic visit in late August 2009. That day, an outside evaluator was accompanying Dr. Novak on her clinical rounds to interview families about their experiences with the West Clinic. When the evaluator asked Kay and Rob what was special about the clinic, both endorsed the ways in which Dr. Novak's explanation tied Michael's pain to aspects of his personality. Rob commented that Dr. Novak had "just pegged him" from Michael's first appointment, and Kay recalled that Rob had called her and said, "It sounds like they've seen Michael before."

That Michael was a type of person that Dr. Novak had seen before suggested to Kay that he was, perhaps, treatable. She explained, "Dr. Novak was able to nail like everything, all the aspects of his personality, how he was feeling, and all of it. I think that was the first moment that Michael kind of finally started to have some hope that if somebody understood it, maybe they could work on [it]." For the Harris family, then, Dr. Novak's personhood diagnostics represented a new way of understanding Michael's pain that promised great hope for therapeutic success.

## EXPLANATORY AMBIVALENCE

To this point, I have argued that Dr. Novak's explanation of pain precasts her patients as highly capable of carrying out a labor-intensive therapeutic protocol by foregrounding their strengths and talents within her diagnostic assessments. I also identified a pragmatic reason for doing so: to shift her patients' therapeutic paradigm. By highlighting the predictive claims of Dr. Novak's explanatory model, I suggested that it offers patients an optimistic view of a future without pain. Furthermore, by tying pain to neurobiological mechanisms, Dr. Novak legitimizes her patients' pain experience and provides a plausible causal narrative. At the same time, however, by implicating personal characteristics, Dr. Novak's personhood diagnostics also projects *backward* to a time well before the pain began.

This temporal structure created certain interpretive difficulties for some of the clinic families, such as that of Zack Morgan, the eleven-year-old CRPS patient introduced at the beginning of this chapter. Zack had developed excruciating foot pain rather suddenly, following a soccer injury. The Morgans consulted several orthopedists and a neurologist before finally being referred to Dr. Novak a few weeks after the injury. Zack had stopped attending his private primary school because his pain cries were too disruptive in the classroom and he was unable to concentrate on his work.

As I reported earlier, at Zack's first clinic appointment, his father, Jon, told me that he was "blown away" by Dr. Novak's suggestion that Zack's smartness and sensitivity were relevant to his diagnosis. I probed deeper into Jon's reaction in an interview conducted two months later. Jon, an entertainment industry executive, spoke extensively about the stigma the family had encountered regarding Zack's CRPS. "People think it's all in his head or that he's emotionally unbalanced," Jon told me. Although Zack's pain had improved significantly, and he had returned to school, the Morgans still faced difficulties with administrators at Zack's school, who refused to admit him for the following school year until they saw how he performed in a mandated summer session.[39] Jon and his wife, Sherri, thought that this was an extreme reaction, since Zack had only missed a few weeks of fifth grade, and a classmate of Zack's with a prolonged medical absence due to a broken arm had been treated much more leniently.

In light of these difficulties, Dr. Novak's explanation of pain offered only tentative relief from the doubts and suspicion that Zack encountered at school and from family and friends. Jon seemed to be of two minds: although Dr. Novak validated Zack's suffering and affirmed that his pain was real, it troubled Jon that her diagnostic explanation also implicated Zack's personhood. As Jon put it, "It's hard to understand the difference between what we know as psychosomatic and a type of personality that would lead to something." Later, he added, "You don't want him to feel like he caused it."

As we talked, Jon struggled to make sense of the difference between "what we know as psychosomatic"—the notion that Zack's pain was "all in his head"—and "a type of personality that would lead to something," Jon's gloss on Dr. Novak's explanation. This ambivalence illustrates how, for patients and families primed to receive psychological explanations for chronic pain, it may be difficult to reconcile the assertion that pain is real and attributable to neurobiological mechanisms with the suggestion that personal characteristics were also involved. For Jon, Dr. Novak's personhood diagnostics seemed to fit with a "misconception" that "it was all in [Zack's] mind to begin with." Such "misconceptions" had significant consequences for Zack. The Morgans attributed what they perceived as the punitive stance of Zack's school administrators to the ambiguous nature of Zack's illness and a belief that the pain was psychosomatic. It did not seem likely to Jon that the administrators would have been more lenient had they been told that Zack's smartness and creativity had kept him absent from school.

Jon's comments illustrate that Dr. Novak's explanatory framework risked being seen as "blaming the victim" by tying pain to personhood and holding patients responsible for treatment outcomes. Social scientists have argued for decades that discourses of individual responsibility divert attention from the structural conditions that shape health.[40] This potential for blame demonstrates that Dr. Novak's explanation did not completely release patients from the harsh moral judgments that have historically pervaded clinical understandings of pain patients.

To the extent that stereotypes gloss over individual variation, they all entail a degree of misrecognition. This darker side of personhood diagnostics is evident in the following observations:

> After Stephanie described her symptoms, Dr. Novak explained that the kids she sees in pain clinic tend to be perfectionists who push themselves hard and excel in school and extracurricular activities. She told the Mortons that these kinds of children have something particular about their neurobiology: the nerve cells make connections easily, and the pain pathways get set up quickly. She explained that this was the downside of being smart, but once Stephanie knows what to do to manage the pain, her smartness and perseverance will help her climb out of it. "All this," Dr. Novak said, "And I haven't even examined you yet. But I know what I'm going to find." (author's field notes, April 13, 2009)

Without raising doubts about Dr. Novak's clinical acuity, the account excerpted above reveals how typecasting can render diagnosis a foregone conclusion. Knowing in advance what one will find can easily lead down a slippery slope in which the patient's problem is explained before it is fully examined. Some parents, like Jon, were wary of such stereotyping, particularly when it revealed clinical biases about the "prototypical patient." One mother was quite critical of the ways in which her daughter had been "put into boxes" by various clinicians (although, notably, not by Dr. Novak) throughout the diagnostic process. For example, she reported that Ted Bridgewater, the team's acupuncturist, had unfairly characterized her daughter as "hypersensitive" because an acupuncture needle had caused her pain.

Tabitha Clarke, a seventeen-year-old girl with all-over body pain, presented a particular challenge in this regard, because she claimed to be a solid B student, the only patient to do so in the time I observed Dr. Novak. Because academic grades were one of Dr. Novak's proxy measures of "smartness" and most of her patients reported receiving straight A's or mostly A's, Tabitha departed from the norm. Nevertheless, because she also indicated that she wrote music, sang, and had had a record deal pending before she got sick, Dr. Novak chose to emphasize these attributes in Tabitha's individualized explanatory account.

> Dr. Novak explained that Tabitha has the neurobiology for someone who is talented in certain areas (i.e., music), and this is why she got "knocked off balance." When the system gets dysregulated, it's like a snowball rolling downhill, getting bigger and bigger because it accumulates more mass. Dr. Novak said that because Tabitha is a very creative, sensitive person, it's not surprising that all this has wreaked havoc on her emotions. Yet it's not emotional—it's real. (author's field notes, April 20, 2009)

Dr. Novak thus maneuvered the challenge posed by individual variability to make Tabitha "fit" the model despite the fact that she did not particularly excel at academics.[41]

This rhetorical dance points to a gap between what we might refer to as "backstage" and "onstage" explanatory models, adopting the sociologist Erving Goffman's dramaturgical metaphor for the theater of everyday life.[42] In the backstage space of clinic meetings, certain patients were less likely to be identified as prototypical patients. In the team meeting following Tabitha's initial appointment, Dr. Novak did not refer to Tabitha's smartness or to her being a typical patient. In clinical interactions, however, any potential differences were erased: all patients effectively embodied the prototype. This was because clinical hermeneutics for reading patients generally afford a great deal of interpretive flexibility and the prototype was pliable enough that all patients could be made to fit the mold.

It also bears mentioning that Dr. Novak was not the only social actor onstage in these interactions. I believe that Michael's receptive stance toward her explanation of pain was authentic, having seen him respond less compliantly in an acupuncture session with Ted Bridgewater later in his treatment. However, Michael had a lot riding on an upbeat clinical performance with Dr. Novak. He had already landed at "the bottom of the funnel," and it was not clear where he would go next if Dr.

Novak were unable (or unwilling) to help him. This underscores that patients and families, too, have a lot invested in strategic clinical performances, especially given the high stakes involved in persuading a doctor that one is *really* in pain.

The discrepancy between backstage and onstage clinical explanations highlights the importance of Kleinman's distinction between the explanatory models employed clinically and those used in professional circles.[43] More broadly, it suggests that the selection of a particular explanatory model is contingent upon the local context of its use. Despite Dr. Novak's insistence in the consultation room that Michael Harris developed pain because he was "smart," in the clinicians' chart room after his first clinic appointment, she hinted that his pain might have been complicated by an undiagnosed condition on the pervasive developmental disorder spectrum, a phenomenon that I discuss further in the next chapter. This subtle sotto voce assertion is exemplary of how Dr. Novak's explanatory framework, as a master diagnostic narrative, diminished various sources of individual difference that might have been relevant to clinical care.

Socioeconomic differences, for example, may influence diagnosis and clinical outcomes, destabilizing the link between a particular patient type and prospective therapeutic efficacy. In this respect, it is important to note that, because most West Clinic patients came from relatively privileged backgrounds, the discourses of achievement and exceptionality that characterized the "prototypical patient" were inflected with other forms of social difference that shaped their educational and extracurricular opportunities, as well as their capacity for self-care. While there is certainly no direct connection between social class and grades, many of the activities that the prototypical patient engaged in were socioeconomically marked. To take advanced placement (AP) classes, for example, one has to attend a high school that offers them, which puts students attending poorly funded public schools (often in inner-city or rural areas) at a distinct disadvantage.[44] Similarly, adolescents who have to work after-school jobs tend to have less time available for sports teams and clubs and related pursuits.

In observing how background assumptions about class shape clinical discourse, it is also worth noting that Dr. Novak's explanatory model was specifically tailored to the achievement orientation typical of middle-class American parents.[45] By validating their children's "smartness," Dr. Novak implicitly transformed their illness into a perverse accomplishment. In one case, I observed a father's expression of grim worry melt away and give way to an expression of pride as he listened to Dr. Novak label his daughter as having a "smart" illness. This reveals how illness, in its relationship to the production of cultural meaning, can become an occasion for articulating social and moral distinctions.

Of course, class-based characterizations are never absolute. Crystal Martinez, who never made it to the West Clinic because of her inadequate health insurance, engaged in just as many extracurricular activities as the West Clinic patients in my study, although she struggled in school. Nevertheless, it seems fair to say that some of the ways in which personhood was understood in this clinical context might overlook the broader relations of inequality that structure both achievement and health in the United States. For instance, although Dr. Novak's explanatory model suggested that therapeutic efficacy hinges on a patient's "smartness," defined as a capacity to change the "patterning in the brain," the use of hypnotherapy clearly privileged patients whose families could afford to pay for a treatment that was rarely covered by insurance.[46] And while explicit class stratification did not emerge among West Clinic patients, the clinic saw very few patients from lower socioeconomic backgrounds to begin with, as Crystal's story reminds us.

These cultural blind spots were undoubtedly influenced by the clinicians' own socioeconomic positioning as clinical professionals. Most remarkable here was their inattentiveness to the homogeneity of the West Clinic's patients as a matter of surprise or concern. What about adolescents who were not gifted? Were they reread or reinvented, along the lines of Tabitha, or were they simply not showing up in the West Clinic at all? Whether Dr. Novak's explanatory model and the clinic's demographics implied that adolescents who were not gifted or privileged did not have this kind of pain or need for such care was not a question that I saw the clinicians engage with. Rather, the prevalence of this particular type of patient was far more likely to inspire an affect-laden paternal pride in their patients' achievements. Although their motives were pure and their care for patients laudable, this elision illustrates that the very ways in which professionals explain illness can reproduce the class biases exemplary of U.S. biomedicine more generally, which powerfully shape the structural determinants of care.

Still, misrecognition takes various forms, and Dr. Novak's approach goes beyond the stereotypes about "psychosomatic" patients in ways that warrant closer attention. Two things in particular stand out about the way that Dr. Novak typecast her patients. First, she employed personhood diagnostics to motivate treatment as well as to assert causal claims. Consequently, rather than evidence of moral weakness, the traits of the prototypical patient were defined as characteristics that would make her more successful in treatment. This future orientation aimed to help the patient to move past questions such as "Am I my illness?" and focus instead on how she might move beyond her illness.

Second, Dr. Novak's explanatory framework relied on a neurobiological register that worked to legitimize the patient's suffering. For Dr. Novak, both pain and personal attributes such as smartness are governed by neurobiological mechanisms. From her perspective, then, while personality may be implicated in pain, it also lies outside of individual control. Accordingly, the person cannot (or should not) be held responsible for it.

Despite these motivations, the ambivalence explored here makes it clear that in an age of "neurochemical selves," where self-understandings are refracted through the biological body, interpreting bodily problems through the lens of neurochemistry does not necessarily free the person from blame.[47] In contrast to the sense of coherence found by the Harris family, Dr. Novak's explanation of pain left the Morgans and other families with a lingering sense of uncertainty regarding responsibility and blame. The point is not that either Jon or the Harrises understood Dr. Novak's explanation superficially. Rather, tying pain to personhood is double-edged and unavoidably morally loaded.

### TRUTH IN DIAGNOSIS

If the diagnostic process is aimed at providing an accurate account of disease to guide treatment decisions, Dr. Novak's explanation of pain raises obvious questions about truth-telling in medicine. When I have presented this work in public forums, some audience members have expressed concerns about the extent to which Dr. Novak might have knowingly misled her patients by suggesting that they were susceptible to chronic pain because they were smart. Others, observing that Dr. Novak's explanatory model functioned something like a placebo in influencing the patient's and family's expectations, have pointed to the ethical challenges involved in the clinical use of placebos. While questions of clinical ethics are important, from an anthropological perspective, a logical starting point to such modes of inquiry is to trouble the dichotomy between deception and truth.

In an eloquent essay on the epistemology of psychosomatic diagnosis, Laurence Kirmayer suggests that the significance of diagnosis is too often reduced to its accuracy, and what this implies for treatment, while neglecting the broader ramifications of diagnostic meaning for healing and self-understanding.[48] Drawing on his extensive clinical experience, Kirmayer points out that psychotherapy is far more concerned with facilitating the creation of meaning than it is with arbitrating truth. He lays out a typology of four forms of clinical truth at stake in psychotherapy: *historical* and *narrative,* which are retrospective truths, meaning that their validity is judged on the basis of their ability to describe past events, and *scientific* and *prescriptive,* prospective forms of truths that are evaluated on their ability to predict future events. Unlike scientific truths, prescriptive truths rely "not on an accurate description of causal mechanisms but on the persuasive power of prediction itself."[49] This is because prescriptive truths are, in Kirmayer's terms, "self-fulfilling prophecies": statements that are not referentially true at the moment of production but that become true as they are incorporated into the patient's worldview.

The notion of prescriptive truth draws attention to the pragmatic meanings of Dr. Novak's explanation of pain and their power to influence patients' recovery. With the concept of prescriptive truth in mind, we might say that Dr. Novak's explanation functions performatively: it becomes true by virtue of saying it is so. From this perspective, more is at stake for the patient than the veracity of Dr. Novak's explanatory model. Specifically, Dr. Novak's explanatory framework offers new possibilities for therapeutic efficacy. As Kirmayer puts it, "The efficacy of prescriptive truth comes from discovering what is possible and from the effects of living life in a new way and so modifying one's own cognitive structures and self-representation as well as eliciting new confirmatory responses from others."[50] Insofar as an everyday pragmatism undergirds many clinical tasks, it is striking that I encountered fewer ethical objections to Dr. Novak's explanatory model when I presented this work to clinical audiences.

Yet if the link between "smart neurons" and chronic pain still seems somewhat absurd, as it has to some of my readers, it may be useful to remember that, within the confines of the clinical encounter, diagnostic rituals can take on a sacred status that resists skeptical questioning. Kleinman cautions that it is not merely the words themselves or the clinician's authority that constitute this sacrality, but rather the powerful, interactive influence of what he calls "clinical reality": "When these explanations are lifted out of the social context they are embedded in, they seem trite and flimsy, because they have lost the compelling meaning that results from their sacred status. They do not amount to much in an academic seminar room. The power of the explanation is precisely that social reality, the culturally constructed clinical world, that functions as the 'real world' for shaman and patient. In this sense, it was the clinical reality, not the clinician, which was effective."[51]

To be clear, I do not mean to suggest that Dr. Novak was engaged in deceptive behavior. Although I have focused on how and why she offered an instrumental account, I also believe that she viewed her explanation as a plausible causal narrative. For Dr. Novak, however, its scientific accuracy was far less important than what her account enabled: a positively valued understanding of pain that helped to motivate responsible, active self-care.

One day, Dr. Novak returned to the chart room after a busy morning with new patients. "I feel like a broken record this morning," she lamented, sinking into a chair. "I'm going to vomit if I use that car metaphor again." By this point, late in my research, Dr. Novak had begun to use the metaphor of a run-down car to describe her patients' ailing bodies as often as she spoke of an electrical engineer who might diagnose their faulty wiring. Laughing, she continued, "I need to go see a rabbi. Rabbis are great with metaphors." As the arbiter of judgments about the reality of pain and the meaning of long-standing suffering, Dr. Novak was no less than a moral broker, which her invocation of Jewish theological authority nicely underscores. If metaphors serve to materialize moral rhetoric, transforming abstract ideas about what is good, valuable, or worthwhile into concrete expressions, then Dr. Novak's inventive explanatory framework, employed in clinical interaction, represents a persuasive moral device as much as a pragmatic therapeutic method.

This chapter has examined the dual-sided potential of a diagnostic ritual that ties unexplained symptoms to a specific type of personhood. Dr. Novak's explanatory framework provides a road map for therapeutic action that renewed the hope of families like the Harrises, while recovering the patient's moral positioning. This prospective orientation, in which the patient's personhood is both an etiological factor and a therapeutic asset, differentiates Dr. Novak's personhood diagnostics from psychosomatic accounts of pain and offers families a more palatable moral framing. By describing hypnotherapy as a way of "rewiring the circuitry," Dr. Novak produced an imaginative, world-changing metaphor that helped to *create* a new reality for Michael, rather than just representing it.[52] At the same time, as we saw with Zack Morgan's case, Dr. Novak's personhood diagnostics reveals certain tensions and fragilities, implicating personal responsibility even as it reframes chronic pain in a positive light. In Dr. Novak's explanatory framing, then, the victim-blaming inherent in characterological explanations of illness is turned on its head: although pain can be linked to personal attributes in a way that may be discrediting, they are nonetheless socially desirable personal attributes. Beyond the individual level of analysis, we have also seen how personhood diagnostics may inadvertently enable the reproduction of class biases in U.S. medicine, even as it provides a persuasive means to alleviate suffering.

By elucidating how Dr. Novak conveyed explanatory models to patients and how these, in turn, mattered for the patient's illness experience, this chapter has illustrated how clinical explanations—and more specifically, characterological ones—can be mobilized as a therapeutic resource. That personhood may be implicated in diagnostic accounts is not a novel idea in anthropological scholarship.[53] What is surprising here, however, is that ascribed forms of clinical personhood may be clinically effective and consonant with cultural values. Thus, while it is clear that diagnostic labeling serves pragmatic clinical functions that come with significant social costs, it would be a mistake to view this typecasting solely in negative terms. Although the diagnostic logic examined here may be reductionistic, it can also be generative of the kinds of subjectivities that patients and their families need to be able to imagine to facilitate healing.

3

# Sticky Brains

I had one patient who had headaches that weren't that severe,
you know. He didn't rate them as being all that severe. But he
said that he was actually suicidal because he couldn't think
about anything else, so he couldn't focus on anything else in
his life, and he couldn't move forward and be productive. So
it wasn't even the severity. So he was actually suicidal, but it
wasn't because of the severity of these headaches. It was
because he couldn't think about anything else.

—Psychologist Nancy Barnes

My *brain* has been terribly "sticky" on a proposal I'm
writing for a conference presentation, and tearing my *brain*
away to even read a news story let alone write about it has
failed some uncountable number of times.

—Dora Raymaker, autism activist

In the preceding chapters, I have illustrated how pediatric pain clinicians,
in conversation with families, employ explanatory frameworks for pain
that rely heavily on neurobiological discourses. They do so primarily to
legitimize mysterious symptoms and disavow psychosomatic models of
pediatric pain, which families might view as dismissive or disbelieving. In
spite of this rhetorical strategy, however, there are many cases in which
clinicians *do* actually believe that, if not exactly "all in your head," in the
sense of being unreal, persistent pain is caused or complicated by a psychological problem. Consequently, the West Clinic pain team sometimes
came to refine their initial explanations with more complex accounts of
the relationship between the neurobiology of pain and individual psychology. In this chapter, I explore a series of cases in which psychological

explanations for the persistence of pain symptoms were folded into the West Clinic's neurobiological explanatory framework. Specifically, I examine a local explanatory model contending that some patients could not get rid of their pain because their brains were "sticky."

In the West Clinic, a widely held explanatory model tied the neurobiology of persistent pain to certain features of pervasive developmental disorder (PDD), such as concrete thinking, an interest in details, and hyperattentiveness. The diagnostic category of PDD was eliminated with the introduction of the fifth version of the American Psychiatric Association's *Diagnostic and Statistical Manual of Mental Disorders* (DSM-5) in May 2013, but at the time of my research, it referred to an umbrella category of five neurodevelopmental disorders, including autism, Asperger syndrome, Rett syndrome, childhood disintegrative disorder, and pervasive developmental disorder not otherwise specified (PDD-NOS).[1] Clinicians used terms such as "sticky brains" and "sticky neurons" to describe the perseverative thoughts and quirky behavior that characterized the sizable minority of the clinic's chronic pain patients who were believed to show signs of PDD, and consequently, did not respond well to treatment. Because of their resistance to standard therapeutic approaches, pain patients suspected of having PDD were considered the most difficult to treat.

As a clinical signifier, the label "sticky brains" does several things. As a metaphor, it represents a set of behavioral and cognitive traits, which I will say more about presently, in terms of a shared neural anatomy presumed to intensify, if not directly cause, the experience of pain. In this sense, and like the concept of "smart neurons," it is a marker of the "neurofication" of human subjectivity.[2] Invoking the brain (and not, for example, the mind or head) in diagnostic reasoning attempts to establish biomedical legitimacy: attributing pain to a "sticky brain" asserts a different sort of claim about the nature of pain than declaring it to be "all in your head." Where the concepts of "sticky brains" and "smart neurons" part company, however, is in the moral valence attached to this peculiar neurobiology. By introducing psychiatric diagnostic criteria, the discourse on sticky brains works to reclassify challenging patients as psychologically abnormal, linking their pain to a preexisting mental disorder.[3] Consequently, whereas the concept of "smart neurons" implicitly reifies pain as real, the concept of "sticky brains" calls the reality of the pain into question. The term "sticky brains" thus encapsulates some of the core tensions—between biological and psychological, psyche and soma—wrapped up in explanations of pain.

## CHRONIC PAIN AND STICKY BRAINS

Pervasive developmental disorders were characterized by three primary features: (1) impairments in communication; (2) impairments in social interaction, and (3) repetitive or stereotyped interests, behaviors, and activities. These features might manifest in various ways, including delayed language development, failure to develop peer relationships, lack of awareness of social conventions, or inflexibility regarding a change in routine.[4] The label PDD could be used as shorthand for PDD-NOS or to refer to the entire spectrum of disorders.[5] In the West Clinic, the term *PDD* was primarily used in a generic sense, to reference the umbrella category. Yet it was also occasionally posed, inaccurately, as a distinctive diagnostic entity in itself.

Discussions of PDD in the West Clinic focused primarily on the third category of diagnostic criteria, which includes repetitive movements, sensory behaviors, and cognitive rigidity. Descriptors such as "sticky brains" and "sticky neurons" linked the perseverative features of PDD to certain attributes of pain patients, such as a tendency to ruminate on pain. The underlying logic of such idioms suggests that these patients got "stuck" on their pain as a result of neurobiological abnormalities. "Sticky brains" was thus a metaphor that indexically linked PDD to chronic pain by highlighting a feature common to both.

Shelly Belkin, a medical student, explained to me how she had learned about this idea: "Dr. Novak talks about this, like how their nervous systems are hard-wired to perseverate on everything. And so when they have a pain experience, they're gonna perseverate on their pain. Like: my foot hurts; my foot hurts; my foot hurts. Their nervous system is, like, *sticky,* and they keep thinking about that." Dr. Petrosian framed this idea particularly evocatively for a seventeen-year-old patient: "All of a sudden you get stuck on an idea. It's like a hangnail on an old sweater—it *sticks.* That's what's going on in your mind."

As these comments suggest, cognitive rigidity and attention difficulties were central to clinical understandings of PDD. The clinical explanatory model tying chronic pain to PDD was based on the premise that people with PDD are at risk for developing intractable pain because of their unusual sensory processing and impaired attention regulation. According to this clinical logic, because many of these patients were also very bright, they were able to compensate for uneven cognitive processing; consequently, their PDD had not been diagnosed. "Sensory processing problems are really common in this population [i.e., people with PDD]," the psychologist Nancy Barnes explained to me. "And they also have many times, um, disordered attentional focus where they perseverate on things. And we know that attentional focus is extremely important in pain perception. And so if you have somebody who has pain and they can't stop thinking about it and focusing on it, we know from functional MRI studies that the area of your brain that lights up in pain gets bigger and bigger and bigger over time. And the stress associated with it is huge because you can't take breaks from it—like people who have more flexible thinking and flexible attentional focus."

Clinicians considered disordered attentional focus to be extremely problematic for chronic pain patients, largely because distraction is widely recognized as an important cognitive coping strategy.[6] For patients with PDD, thoughts of pain were presumed to be literally inescapable. "It's harder for them to distract themselves or to find things to distract themselves," Nina Herrera, the clinical coordinator, told me. "They don't know how to do that." The prevailing clinical wisdom thus held that patients with PDD did not respond well to traditional therapeutic interventions because their pain produced an enormous cognitive burden.

It is important to stress that this understanding of the relationship between chronic pain and PDD was a local one; to my knowledge, there is no empirical basis for this relationship in the research literature.[7] In fact, *reduced* sensitivity to pain has been more commonly reported among children with autism, though some have suggested that a lower pain response in this population may be better explained by different modes of pain expression than by pain insensitivity.[8] Given the local specificity of this explanatory model, it is important to ask what "sticky brains" *do* in the everyday talk of the clinic. As we have already seen, in the West Clinic, neurobiological discourse provided a powerful frame for understandings of personhood. Yet the brain itself, as a material object, remained curiously absent from clinical discussions. Clinicians did not identify structural or functional brain differences associated with stickiness, nor did they assign patients whom they suspected of having PDD to particular treatment options—though they often invoked "stickiness" as an explanation for why treatments did not work.

Consequently, characterizing certain patients as "sticky" worked less to bring previously undiagnosed neurodevelopmental disorders to light than it did to explain and justify why certain adolescents were so difficult to treat. In the anthropologist Rebecca Lester's terms, clinical discourse on PDD corresponded to "soft" diagnosis, or "the working models clinicians use in assessing what is causing the difficulty," rather than "hard" diagnosis—"diagnosis according to standardized criteria like the DSM."[9] In soft diagnosis, there is often a conflation of therapeutic and bureaucratic goals: the diagnosis may diffuse practical clinical problems more than it improves actual treatment options. In this setting, then, PDD functioned as a diagnostic black box: clinicians did not need to understand its DSM history or its nosological complexity to make pragmatic use of its explanatory power for the routine tasks of patient care.

While categorizations such as "sticky brains" are basic to institutional life, classificatory systems hide as much as they reveal.[10] Here, I am not principally concerned with the disputed ontology of neurological stickiness—that is, with whether these patients did or did not have PDD in a "hard" diagnostic sense. Instead, I aim to illuminate the pragmatic function of clinical discourse on stickiness and the relational complexities it necessarily elides.

### INDEXICAL MARKERS OF STICKINESS

Encounters with stickiness sometimes began even before face-to-face meetings with patients. Parents and adolescents were routinely asked to complete lengthy surveys that were mailed to the family's home prior to their first appointment in the clinic. The questionnaires elicited basic demographic information, as well as information about the patient's medical background, treatment history, and medications. They also included psychological measures that Dr. Novak used in her clinical research. Before Dr. Novak or Dr. Petrosian entered the examination room and introduced themselves to a new family, a researcher collected the questionnaires from each patient and one of his or her parents. In keeping with a clinical ideology of pain management that suggested that talking about pain draws attention to the body and sometimes exacerbates how it feels, the questionnaire procedure enabled physicians to glean a great deal of medical information before meeting the patients and saved valuable clinical time. But respondents' questionnaires also afforded a sort of projective lens onto patient and parent personalities: before meeting a new patient, Dr. Novak and Dr. Petrosian regularly scanned the intake questionnaires in search of clues about the type of people they would soon be meeting.

To this end, the page-length diagrams of the front and back of the human body, on which patients and parents were instructed to indicate the location of the pain, served as a striking signpost in the clinical hermeneutics of reading patients. Early in my research, I encountered a seventeen-year-old girl who had color-coded and shaded her pain diagram in exquisite detail. Both figures, front and back, were covered in vibrant hues of purple, red, and green, signifying her full-body pain. The clinicians immediately viewed such painstaking attention to detail on the pain diagram exercise as indicative of the intense bodily focus believed to characterize patients with PDD. As it turned out, the patient had been diagnosed with Asperger syndrome many years prior to her visit in the pain clinic; she was one of two such patients with a previously diagnosed pervasive developmental disorder who came to the clinic during the course of my study. In another case I observed, a ten-year-old boy had covered the entire lower extremities of the figure on his pain diagram with carefully drawn X's, prompting the clinicians in the chart room to suggest the possibility that he had PDD.

Occasionally, the very act of filling out the intake questionnaire was itself laden with diagnostic meaning. Once, a new patient of Dr. Novak's, an eleven-year-old boy, came to the clinic without having filled out his questionnaire. While this in itself was not that uncommon, since families often forgot or ran out of time, Tim Dupont, the research assistant assigned to collect the questionnaires before the family's meeting with Dr. Novak, had a very difficult time coaxing the boy to answer the questions. Tim reported that the boy would circle two or three responses for a single item and refuse to correct his answers and complete the questionnaire. He also refused to sign the assent form that would permit his data to be used for clinical research. When Tim relayed these difficulties back to Dr. Novak in the chart room, she chuckled, "Oh, he *is* PDD!"

I call these projective behaviors and traits—drawing a pain diagram with painstaking detail and obstinacy toward clinical protocols—*indexical markers of PDD* because of the ways in which they triggered clinical heuristics for dealing with "difficult" patients. While these indexical markers were not foolproof signs of who might come to embody the PDD label, they nevertheless provided clinicians with meaningful clues about challenging patient behavior. Backstage discussions in the West Clinic were rife with references to such indexical markers. For example, Dr. Novak once told a medical student working with her that whenever she saw a "computer geek," she wondered whether he or she was on the PDD spectrum. She counseled the student to follow up on such questions by asking about whether the patient had ever collected anything, because children with PDD engage in a restricted range of activities due to their perseverations. "Once they develop an interest in something, they tend to stick with it," Dr. Novak explained. Here, interests in computers and collections served as indexical markers of stickiness that prompted specific clinical heuristics. Dr. Novak's explanation—"they tend to *stick* with it"—indexically ties her patients' perseverative behavior to the specific neurobiology—that is, "sticky" brains—presumed to underlie it.

Dr. Novak and Dr. Petrosian routinely probed for specific indexical markers of PDD in clinic intake appointments. In Michael Harris's intake appointment, for example, Dr. Novak asked his father, Rob, "Is Michael argumentative? So that if he has a point he will stick with it." When Rob nodded his head, Dr. Novak inquired about whether Michael collected anything. Michael responded that he had a collection of eighty shot glasses and was running out of space to store them. Dr. Novak went on to ask Rob about whether Michael had ever experienced sensitivity to clothes or certain textures, to which Michael replied that he couldn't stand walking around without socks. Such sensory sensitivity signaled yet another indexical marker of PDD.

It is important to emphasize, however, that indexical markers were not in themselves determinative of PDD.[11] In one teaching interaction, Dr. Novak instructed Ava Thomas, a medical student, to probe for PDD when taking the case history of a seventeen-year-old male with testicular pain. Dr. Novak had noted diagnoses of obsessive compulsive disorder (OCD) and attention deficit/ hyperactivity disorder (ADHD) on the patient's intake questionnaire, and she explained to Ava that many patients with testicular pain have a "sticky" nervous system and that Asperger syndrome can masquerade as conditions such as OCD or ADHD. She primed Ava to inquire about separation anxiety, collections, and school performance. When Ava returned from collecting the patient's history, she relayed that the patient had maintained poor eye contact throughout their interaction and displayed some PDD-like characteristics, such as perseveration. Yet after Dr. Novak examined the patient herself, she told Ava that she thought his anxiety and depression were confusing the diagnostic picture. Dr. Novak did not, in the end, think that the patient had PDD.[12]

Outside of these teaching encounters, indexical markers of PDD were most commonly employed in the weekly team meetings. For example, when Maura Roberts, a clinical psychology postdoctoral fellow, told the team that she had turned off the lights in her office because of a patient's migraine headaches and light sensitivity, Charlotte LeFevre, the team hypnotherapist, exclaimed, "He's on the spectrum!" Similarly, the team discussed another patient whose father had a history of chronic pain and would avoid his wife and daughter by isolating himself in a dark room. When Dr. Novak heard this, she averred that this father had Asperger syndrome.

On another occasion, a medical student referred to a new patient's "PDD-like traits" and described his interest in maps and timetables and his desire to be a pilot. Dr. Petrosian leveraged a similar cluster of traits toward diagnostic insight when he characterized a fourteen-year-old patient as "into maps, airplanes, and weather." Dr. Novak responded promptly, "So he's Asperger's," to which Dr. Sterling, the team's psychiatrist, mused with feigned naïveté, "Doctor, whatever makes you say that?" Such knowing exchanges demonstrate the physicians' pragmatic understanding of the rich semiotic loading of maps, airplanes, and weather. By alluding to such indexical markers of PDD, team members reflected and constructed an epistemic culture in which peculiar habits and everyday objects were assumed to offer rich diagnostic meaning, if not necessarily hard evidence.

## FAMILIES ENCOUNTERING STICKINESS

While Dr. Novak repeatedly described Michael Harris as "PDDish" and "on the PDD spectrum" in the team meetings, she never mentioned PDD to the Harris family. Unlike "smart neurons," which featured prominently in onstage clinical rhetoric, clinicians typically limited their use of the sticky label to the clinic's backstage spaces, choosing euphemisms instead in onstage contexts—"You know, I think it's possible that his neurological wiring is such that he tends to see things concretely," as the child and family therapist Rebecca Hunter put it—until they had developed rapport with the family. Michael's case demonstrates that "smart neurons" and "sticky brains" could coexist as explanatory tropes in individual cases, because they served different rhetorical purposes and catered to different audiences. Clinicians tended to avoid PDD talk with families, not only because most families were both familiar with and afraid of the autism spectrum, but also because psychiatric language and explanations were so morally loaded in this clinical domain.

On several occasions, however, sticky brains and PDD were raised with patients and families early on. One such patient was Mark Siegel, the fourteen-year-old boy who developed CRPS following a boogie-boarding injury. At Mark's first clinic appointment, Julie handed Dr. Petrosian a lengthy list of the treatments, physicians, and medications that Mark had tried and told him, "We heard you were the best."[13] Julie was particularly concerned about Mark's high blood pressure, which she attributed to his pain. Now that it had affected his heart, Julie explained, they were determined to get Mark some relief. "And nobody in this city has been able to help him," Julie lamented. "So you feel the pressure?" her husband, Micah, asked. "I like it," Dr. Petrosian said, nodding. "I like that you like it," Julie replied. The laughter that followed only partially eased the mounting tension. Julie's strategic self-presentation was bolder and more forthright than that of most parents I observed in similar clinical scenes.[14]

Julie indicated that Mark, whom she described a "gifted kid," taking mainly honors courses in his ninth-grade year, had been taking the drug Pamelor for attention deficit disorder for the past six years.[15] Mark reported that his hobbies included the Internet, Tetris, "TV, and "watching airplanes"—he was a member of the largest aviation web site and tracked flight paths online. Evidencing his PDD heuristic in practice, Dr. Petrosian probed for additional indexical markers of PDD by asking Mark whether he had ever been fascinated by maps (yes) or trains (no). During the course of the consultation, Dr. Petrosian told Mark, "One of the major problems here, you have too good of a memory." This explanation was consistent with the clinical model of sticky brains.

At the end of the appointment, Dr. Petrosian sent Mark home with a prescription for the pain medication Neurontin, some anesthetic patches for topical pain relief, and referrals to the pain team's physical therapist and hypnotherapist. He also suggested to Mark and his father that they follow up with Mark's current psychiatrist, explaining that ADD might have been a mistaken diagnosis, and that Mark might instead have PDD. As he put it: "ADD-type kids, their attention can't focus on one thing, right? 'Oh, those shoes are cool, no, I like Dad's shoes better, lemme grab that.' Y'know, with or without hyperactivity. PDD kids are more like, 'My pain.' And then you can say, 'Come on, there's a fire behind you.' 'Yeah, but my left elbow hurts.' 'Come on, we're getting nuked here.' 'Yeah, but my elbow hurts.' You see what I mean?"

Dr. Petrosian's diagnostic speculation claimed little explanatory purchase with the Siegel family. Julie, who had missed this explanation because she left the appointment early to attend a business meeting, was livid when I caught up with her the next day. She told me that she had spent thousands of dollars on the neuropsychologist who had diagnosed Mark's ADD and was outraged by the suggestion that Mark might instead have PDD.

At their next meeting, aware of his misstep, Dr. Petrosian tried to reassure the Siegels that a psychiatry referral was "not to say it's in [his] head," but rather, "to make sure that [the] parallel obstacle's being cleared." But if therapeutic pathways contribute to diagnostic meaning, then pursuing a psychiatric evaluation very clearly suggested to Mark and his parents that Dr. Petrosian believed that Mark's pain was in fact "in his head." By suggesting that Mark's long-standing pain might be explained by a secondary disorder that predated his boogie-boarding injury, Dr. Petrosian invoked a more complex explanation for Mark's pain—one that the Siegel family viewed as a threat to Mark's legitimacy. Referral to a psychiatrist suggested a new therapeutic trajectory whose future course was much less certain and much less likely to bring quick relief, while at the same time shifting the burden of care.

Although Julie was cordial to Dr. Petrosian in this onstage interaction, in a phone conversation I had with her after Mark's second clinic appointment, she told me that she was extremely dissatisfied and did not plan to return to the West Clinic. Mark's long-term psychiatrist, Dr. Middleton, disagreed with Dr. Petrosian's assessment, she said. "Therapy would be worthless," she told me. "We need to get him out of pain." Having already spent thousands of dollars on psychiatric evaluations, she did not want to spend more pursuing a diagnosis of PDD. She added angrily: "I don't give a shit if [Mark] has a sticky brain! If you don't fit in [Dr. Petrosian's] box, he has no idea what to do with you!" A few weeks later, Julie informed me that another doctor had told her that "the 'PDD shit' is wrong when it comes to CRPS—it's just bad luck."

. . .

Some parents reacted more favorably than Julie Siegel to allegations of stickiness. Dr. Novak recounted one case in a team meeting in which she raised the possibility of PDD at a first clinical meeting and the parents responded receptively. The patient was Abraham Rubin, the eleven-year-old boy who had refused to provide assent to participate in Dr. Novak's clinical research. Abraham had been diagnosed with juvenile idiopathic arthritis in his left knee, which had been relatively well controlled. Recently, however, he had begun to complain about pain elsewhere in his body, and his pediatrician had diagnosed him with fibromyalgia. Abraham had also been diagnosed with a learning disability, and a neuropsychologist had suggested that he attend a special school, but the Rubins, who were Orthodox Jews, wanted him to be able to attend a Jewish day school.

When Dr. Novak examined Abraham, she found no trigger points—sensitive spots in the muscle tissue that serve as diagnostic criteria for fibromyalgia. She asked the Rubins if Abraham was argumentative, if he had difficulty with transitions, if he was particular about his clothing, and if they felt as if they had to "walk on eggshells" around him. They responded affirmatively to all of these questions. When Dr. Novak asked if Abraham had any collections, they said no, but they did admit to his having "keepsakes," which, it became clear, were essentially the same thing.

According to Dr. Novak, she next described PDD, and "everything fit." Abraham did not fit the criteria for fibromyalgia; his aches and pains were just "perseverations." The Rubins had attributed Abraham's irritability to his pain, when really it was the opposite: his pain could be attributed to his stickiness. According to Dr. Novak, the Rubins were relieved, and welcomed her diagnosis enthusiastically. Despite consulting multiple physicians, no one had connected his symptoms in a way that made sense. Dr. Novak concluded, to the team: "it's a non-pain diagnosis."

In general, Dr. Novak was far less likely than Dr. Petrosian to use the PDD label with families at a first clinic meeting, preferring instead to focus on establishing a relationship with the family and refer the patient to Rebecca Hunter for a psychological evaluation or to neuropsychological testing outside the West Clinic. With this in mind, Dr. Novak's successful deployment of the PDD label with the Rubin family appears all the more striking, reflecting a carefully honed clinical insight that enabled her to sort out, on the ground, the families that might respond to this language receptively. Dr. Novak's years of clinical experience likely account for why she was more successful than Dr. Petrosian in broaching PDD with families.

Another mother, whose daughter had already been diagnosed with a pervasive developmental disorder, similarly welcomed the "sticky" diagnosis. Lori Donovan had been convinced that there must be a connection between her daughter Cameron's migraine headaches and her long-term autism diagnosis, but the neurologists she had consulted did not support this view. So when Dr. Novak told Lori that she saw this kind of pain problem "with much more frequency in kids who had a PDD background," Lori felt validated. As she put it, "I really liked having that missing link filled in. You know, that was just really bugging me somehow. And to have somebody who understood how this fit into our medical history is, you know, just um, made me much more confident in everything that she was telling us."

Despite these optimistic cases, many of the pain team's clinicians recounted considerable family resistance to talking about PDD. However, parental resistance only served to strengthen clinical convictions about the very phenomena that parents called into question. This was because parental resistance was often interpreted as a sign that the parents themselves were "sticky." That is, an important presumption of the clinical model of sticky brains was that stickiness ran in families.

## STICKY FAMILIES

In pediatric settings, where parents and children tend to share the patient role, it may be just as likely for stickiness to be attributed to parents as to the patients themselves. It was not uncommon for clinicians to draw diagnostic inferences about parents from their reports or behavior in the clinic, although these remained limited to backstage clinical discussions. Once, in a team meeting, Dr. Novak described a consultation with a new patient in which she reported to have "nearly diagnosed the boy through his father." Everything she described about pain and sticky neurology elicited a nod of sympathetic agreement from the father, who suffered from long-term chronic neck pain and "seemed PDD." "Oh yeah, that describes me," the father had reportedly said. Likewise, explaining the value of having parents present for clinical consultations, the medical student Shelly Belkin said, "Dr. Novak would say, like you have a kid who has like PDD—pervasive developmental disorder. And she'd go, well, I can tell which parent has it. Dad has it. . . . it is great when you can have the whole family there, for sure."

Sticky families presented clinical challenges on several fronts, not the least of which was their propensity to consume a disproportionate share of clinical resources. Dr. Novak told me about one father who was "very needy," with whom she had spent "an enormous amount of time." He would call or e-mail frequently, insisting that he needed to speak with her directly, refusing to share his concerns with Nina Herrera, her clinical assistant. Once, he showed up in the clinic unscheduled to speak with her about a pressing matter. "You know, I don't dislike him but there are certain behaviors that can be very annoying," Dr. Novak admitted.

In interviews, I typically asked clinicians to describe a patient who had been a particular challenge to help. On several occasions, this prompt elicited a discussion of a family in which multiple members appeared to show signs of PDD. My interview with Rebecca Hunter was particularly illuminating in this regard. Rebecca had been working with the family of Ted Lewis, an eighteen-year-old with chronic headaches and "extreme Asperger's, not acknowledged by the family." According to Rebecca, Ted "basically barricades himself in his room and never comes out." Rebecca had been meeting with Ted's parents for several years. Ted was unable to come to her office himself due to his sensory sensitivity, which she attributed to his PDD. As she told me, "'I can't have Ted in here because [of] the decibel level in the room . . . he hears the different amplifications, and . . . he's really, really extreme Asperger's." Rebecca suspected that the father had Asperger syndrome as well.

The greatest challenge for Rebecca was getting the Lewis family to follow a behavioral incentive plan to encourage Ted to leave his bedroom and go to school. Rebecca indicated that the parents "have no ability to co-parent—no ability to follow through on anything." She explained: "What happens is, the parents will come in, and I'll like go through the whole parenting thing with them, and then they'll disappear for four months. And then they'll come back in a crisis, we'll spend the whole session recapping what's gone on for four months, and then I won't hear from them." Much of Rebecca's frustration seemed to focus on the father's unwillingness to accept the diagnosis of Asperger syndrome. Although Rebecca had arranged for Ted to undergo neuropsychological testing and the tests had suggested that he did indeed have Asperger syndrome, she noted, "The mom kind of understood; the dad wouldn't hear any of it." She had given them books to read explaining the diagnosis, but "Mom will flag the pages in the books I give them and give them to Dad and he won't even look at them."

That Rebecca was quick to contrast this father's and mother's responses demonstrates her belief that some of the father's resistance emanated from his own stickiness. Her comments also illustrate why work with patients suspected of having PDD became complexly sticky: if a patient exhibited sticky thinking, the odds were good that a parent would as well. This view of stickiness as hereditary corresponded both with some of the more psychodynamically oriented clinical ideologies, which held that pain symptoms tend to cluster in families due to learned behavior, and with popular understandings of the genetics of PDD. That PDD was seen to run in families suggested that adolescents were "difficult" patients because they hailed from "difficult" families.

Rebecca's comments underscore the intricacies of offering clinical care in a context in which therapy was almost always entangled with complex family relations. Dr. Petrosian compared the West Clinic to his private practice, noting, "Every single case has the family involved. Whereas for [my other clinic] they might not be as involved or affected or afflicted." I asked how that affected his job. "Makes it tougher," he said. "You're responsible for the whole unit. The family unit. The household unit."

In working with "sticky" families, troubles arose not only around diagnostic acceptance, but also around soliciting the family's cooperation to pursue a particular therapeutic path. Cecilia Rubio, a medical student, recounted another challenging case that illustrates how "sticky" parents could create obstacles to treatment. She spoke of a patient who Dr. Novak believed had PDD. The patient had undergone neuropsychological testing, which identified deficits in neurosensory integration, a hallmark of PDD. In describing the difficulties of the case, however, Cecilia highlighted the mother's behavior: "And, um, Mom was very PDD also. She was . . . just really stuck on that diagnosis and she wanted to know exactly what was causing it . . . how it was gonna be treated." According to Cecilia, this mother did her own online research and "wrote, like, several e-mails a week explaining what new things she'd learned." Yet why, we might ask, should it be so surprising for a mother to insist on knowing what was causing her child's illness and how it would be treated—or to be "stuck" on the diagnosis, as Cecilia put it? Perhaps more to the point: what is to be gained by ascribing pathology to parents?

• • •

At the final team meeting in which Mark Siegel's case was discussed, before Julie cut ties with the clinic, Dr. Petrosian described a series of telephone conversations he had had with her in which she had pressured him to prescribe two specific drugs. Mark was not responding to the Neurontin that Dr. Petrosian initially prescribed, and Julie was worried that it was interfering with his schoolwork. Several West Clinic patients, including Mark, noted that they had difficulty concentrating while taking Neurontin. This side effect complements the clinic's folk model of stickiness in interesting ways: if patients got "stuck" on pain at least in part due to disordered attentional focus, it made sense that a drug designed to disrupt attention to pain would have similar cognitive effects in other domains. In fact, Dr. Petrosian interpreted Mark's failure to experience the intended effects of Neurontin as further evidence of his PDD, telling the family at their second clinic visit that Neurontin was the "bread and butter" treatment for CRPS, but that it had no effect on PDD.

Discouraged by Mark's experience with Neurontin, Julie had inquired among her pharmaceutical industry colleagues about possible pharmacological treatments. She subsequently pressed Dr. Petrosian to prescribe two specific medications for Mark that had been recommended by her contacts: a steroid to address the inflammation around his elbow, and Ultram, an opioid analgesic used to treat moderate to severe pain. In addition, Julie e-mailed Nina Herrera to say that if she did not hear back from Dr. Petrosian, she would ask her neighbor, a high-ranking hospital administrator, for a referral.[16] "She's the thunder factor in this," Dr. Petrosian concluded. Dr. Novak asked whether Julie "was PDD," and Dr. Petrosian replied, "Heck yeah!"

After some initial resistance, Julie persuaded Dr. Petrosian to write the prescription for the Ultram, but not for the steroid. Meanwhile, she refused to bring Mark in for a consultation with Dr. Sterling, the team's psychiatrist, and to schedule a family therapy session with Rebecca Hunter. The family's contact with the clinic petered out soon after Mark finished the Ultram.

The attribution of stickiness to Julie resulted from her insistence on particular pharmaceutical treatments. What this explanation masks, however, is that criticizing Julie made it easier for the clinicians to rationalize Mark's failed treatment. This clinical logic suggested that if only Julie had followed the recommended course of action rather than introducing her own requests, they might have been able to help Mark. Without parental "buy-in," treatment had no hope of succeeding.

Yet the clinicians' willingness, not only to blame parents for therapeutic failures, but also to *diagnose* them suggests that something more was at stake. It is one thing to employ a clinical metaphor like stickiness, which sharpens the meaning of a "difficult" parent's behavior; it is quite another to apply a DSM diagnosis, which implies pathological, and not merely problematic, behavior. Parental diagnosis implied that clinical problems were deeply entrenched in longer temporal trajectories, which could take years, or even generations, to unravel. Depicting PDD as a multigenerational phenomenon thus made it appear all the more intractable. Furthermore, diagnoses have far greater clinical potential than do metaphors, and they are endowed with greater independent agency. The label PDD, even if only uttered behind closed doors, might make a clinician approach a new parent-patient pair suspiciously, and could affect the types of therapeutic strategies offered. Functionally, then, a "soft" diagnosis of PDD could take on a life of its own, even if it had not been officially sanctioned.[17]

## STICKY ENCOUNTERS AND IDIOMS OF DISTRESS

In an influential article published in 1981, the anthropologist Mark Nichter introduced the term *idioms of distress* to describe the culturally constituted expressive modes through which people express distress.[18] Nichter urged anthropologists to move away from fixed diagnostic categories to attend instead to the contextual meanings of illness and suffering and the culturally elaborated interactional styles through which distress is expressed. Drawing inspiration from this call, I suggest that "stickiness" functioned as an idiom of distress that encapsulated the difficulties of living with chronic pain. Yet whose distress is in question? The scholars who have employed Nichter's terminology have invariably focused on patients.[19] In this case, however, I have come to see stickiness as a metaphor for the difficulties of the clinical encounter, which may just as easily (though admittedly differently) burden each party in a therapeutic interaction. Stickiness, from this perspective, may be seen as an interpretive lens from which to view clinical difficulties more generally.

By broadening the "idioms of distress" framework in this way, I acknowledge that clinicians also get stuck. It is quite telling in this regard that when I asked Dr. Novak about the benefits of working on an interdisciplinary team, she replied, "I really appreciate the input [about] the patients I'm stuck on . . . stuck about, or confused about, um, just ventilation and support. For difficult parents." Striking here is Dr. Novak's replacement of "patients" with "parents" in referencing what makes her "stuck."

In the discourse on "sticky brains" employed in the West Clinic, clinical, relational problems were transmuted into neurological defects. This discursive framing transformed a shared, collective burden into a concrete personal problem. When we consider that idioms of distress are often seen as rhetorical tools for framing psychological complaints in somatic terms to bolster their legitimacy, the neurological language makes sense.[20] Yet where should we locate stickiness: in the brain or the social world? Autism scholars have asked various versions of this question in slightly different formats.[21] In the case of chronic pain, locating stickiness in a patient's brain as opposed to the social world presupposes a very different sort of intervention. The discourse of stickiness shifts the locus of blame for diagnostic and therapeutic complexity from the clinic to the patient herself. This shifting of blame mitigates threats to clinical efficacy and helps to explain why the PDD label was sometimes used in backstage clinic spaces, even if it was not explicitly employed in dialogue with families.

Yet what this discourse elides is that stickiness might just as easily describe the failures of biomedicine to address the needs of these patients (and their families). In other words, by leveraging diagnostic insights about "difficult" patients, clinicians may misrecognize deeply entrenched difficulties whose sources are located far outside of individual pathology. As Nadia Agarwal, a medical student, suggested to me, it is extraordinarily challenging to treat patients who rarely seem to get better: "If they've seen so many other clinicians and have tried a lot of other treatment options . . . it just signals it's a difficult case. And if every case is difficult like that, it can be really stressful to . . . never have a case where it's very easy to manage." Rationalizing treatment resistance through the discourse of stickiness was one way of alleviating this burden and making difficult cases easier to handle.

It is important, however, not to overlook the fact that for all of its pragmatic purposes, the idiom of stickiness resonated with some patients and families at a fundamental phenomenological level. When I asked twelve-year-old Cameron Donovan what Dr. Novak had told her about her pain, she said, "She explained it like, you know, [a] very simple way. That I sort of had a sticky brain and where like other people um, they, like- other people you know, would get over it, I- it continued to stay there. Which I kind of already knew." When I asked Cameron how she knew this, she replied, "Well, because I *felt* it." For Cameron, who developed what her mother described as an "obsessive interest" in memorizing gymnastics routines as her headaches intensified, "stickiness" captured an inexplicable quality of her experience of perseveration.

Even Julie Siegel, despite her serious complaints, suggested that she did in fact believe that something akin to what Dr. Petrosian called stickiness affected Mark's pain. Once, when reflecting on Mark's therapeutic engagement, Julie alluded to some of the characteristics of "sticky" thinking that the clinical ideology tied to PDD. Mark had been asking Julie persistently about some therapeutic alternatives that they might be able to pursue for his pain. Finally, Julie told Mark to "take a deep breath," and then, turning to me, explained, "I mean, that's the other thing, is, his brain is just—he doesn't rest his brain ever. He's just constantly going." She continued, "I mean, he wakes up in the morning and he, first thing he says to us is, 'I wanna do this, I want you to call this doctor, I want this done, I want you to make sure this gets done.'"

It is striking that in referring to Mark's hyperattentiveness and extreme focus, Julie invoked some of the very same qualities that Dr. Petrosian had used in labeling Mark as "sticky." His tendency to wake up in the morning with a clear, pressing agenda likewise relates to the quality of perseveration that Dr. Petrosian had categorized as a defining feature of PDD. For all of her objections, then, Julie also found Mark behaviorally sticky. It was not necessarily the description that she objected to, but rather its complex entailments.

## DISAPPEARING OBJECTS

Some readers no doubt will wonder what to make of the clinical discourse on sticky brains and whether the association between chronic pain and PDD holds descriptive validity. However, the point of my research (as for many clinically oriented anthropological projects) was not to determine whether these patients did or did not have PDD. Instead, the purpose was to critically analyze how clinicians manage therapeutic difficulties. In adopting this approach, I have followed Rebecca Lester, who, in her study of how clinicians treating eating disorders talk about borderline personality disorder (BPD), claimed to have been "less interested in whether BPD exists a priori" than in how the category of BPD enabled clinicians to confront certain ethical dilemmas in patient care.[22]

And yet, whether or not a relationship exists between chronic pain and a set of cognitive and behavioral traits that we might colloquially call "sticky," PDD itself no longer exists—at least not within psychiatric nosology. The ontological politics of this reclassification raise an interesting question for anthropologists: how do we think and write about something that technically does not exist? In the anthropology of psychiatry, this question is often framed in terms of psychiatric objects that do not exist there (and, implicitly, yet).[23] But in this case, the issue is not one of globalizing forms of knowledge, but of the effects of changes in diagnostic categories on how we conceptualize clinical objects.

Although my research had long been completed by the time DSM-5 was released, the disappearance of PDD from it only confirmed for me the ontological slipperiness of "stickiness." Unevenness in the application of criteria for Asperger syndrome and PDD-NOS was cited as a major reason for the revision of the PDD category,[24] and this concern resonated with my experience in the West Clinic, where wielding the label seemed to confuse as much as it clarified. While I cannot comment directly on how the clinicians themselves responded to this change, which was rolled out several years after my fieldwork ended, I wonder whether it even registered a shift in their deeply pragmatic practice. The discourse of stickiness had always reflected a behind-the-scenes logic more than an institutionalized nosology. For the anthropologist, however, the removal of PDD from the DSM raised the question of whether there ever had been anything inside the West Clinic's diagnostic black box. An enduring lesson of psychiatric anthropology has been the idea that mental disorders are not concrete things but, rather, unstable categories, shape-shifters that bend and sway with the local clinical and cultural context. In this case, then, analyzing something that officially no longer exists has brought to the foreground how the production of scientific knowledge, an always ongoing and emergent process, unsettles established frames of inquiry and challenges categories already in play.

The disappearance of PDD from the DSM also raises questions about the gendered nature of PDD. For more than a decade, the eminent autism researcher Simon Baron-Cohen has argued that some of the features of autism—primarily obsessions and repetitive behaviors—may signal an extreme form of the normal male brain. The extreme-male-brain theory of autism proposes that autism lies at one end of a continuum of populationwide sex differences in the capacity for empathizing and systematizing: people with autism have a below-average capacity for empathy and an above-average interest in systems, giving them an extreme form of the "normal" male brain.[25]

While the extreme-male-brain-theory of autism has been challenged by feminist scholars and within the medical community, the contraction of the PDD category at least raises the possibility that some cases of what was formerly known as PDD might lie toward one end of a normal spectrum of gendered behavior rather than constituting pathology. Many of the behaviors flagged in the West Clinic as indexical markers of PDD—such as Mark Siegel's interest in aviation—were stereotypically male, and male patients, likewise, were much more likely to be labeled "sticky."[26] The possibility that indexical markers of PDD might instead reflect an extreme display of maleness (in the U.S. cultural context) underscores the extent to which psychiatric judgments hinge on adjudications of normality.

Above all, the disappearance of PDD—and the politics underlying it—makes it clear that diagnosis is an ongoing, negotiated process that reveals the pragmatic needs of clinicians and patients as much as it settles the facts about an illness. The debate surrounding the removal of Asperger syndrome and PDD-NOS from the DSM highlights the contingent nature of psychiatric categories and the sociocultural forces that transform them over time. What makes the social life of the PDD category particularly fascinating in the context of the West Clinic, however, is that it is entangled with another category whose ontological status is equally fuzzy.

## ALL IN THE BRAIN?

While interesting in their own right, the clinical heuristics for PDD were especially remarkable for how they were brought to bear on pain. By suggesting that a preexisting neurodevelopmental disorder was responsible for the patient's failure to respond to standard treatment, the discourse on sticky brains dramatically altered the meaning of chronic pain. There is, of course, a long-standing tradition of explaining chronic pain in terms of psychological disorder: the term "psychogenic" pain, although it has since been discarded for multidimensional causal models, was long used to describe pain caused or prolonged by psychological factors. In this case, however, because of the rhetorical power of the brain in explaining mental disorder, individual psychology was invoked in a different way than by such psychosomatic models. That is, pain might not be "all in your head" but rather "all in your brain."

Neurobiological explanations for psychiatric conditions are typically exculpatory, insofar as localizing disorder in the brain tends to free the self from blame.[27] Yet introducing psychiatric explanations in a pain clinic is highly morally charged and tends to arouse patients' suspicions, even when these explanations are couched in neurobiological terms. The case of sticky brains thus illustrates that neurobiological explanatory discourse does not always work in the service of biomedical legitimization.

It also highlights some of the unsettling consequences of splitting the self from the brain. In chapter 2, we saw how Dr. Novak characterized "smart neurons" as an important therapeutic resource. This explanation frames the brain-self split in a positive light: neurons are the self's ally in the fight against pain. In contrast, the explanatory model of pain that Dr. Petrosian offered the Siegel family suggested that although Mark was smart, his pain resisted treatment because his brain was "sticky." In this case, then, the brain obstructs the self's quest for recovery. The possibility of stickiness thus points to a fundamental tension within the clinic's explanatory discourse, which imaginatively cast patients as agentive actors capable of rewiring their neural circuitry, even as it endowed their brains with an independent agency that might conflict with the self's actions and desires.

In light of this tension, the discourse on stickiness offered some patients and families a welcome conceptual language for understanding social difference and translating it into a neurobiological frame. This was certainly the case with Cameron Donovan and Abraham Rubin and their families. For others, like the Siegel family, however, accepting the label of stickiness was tantamount to acknowledging that chronic pain might, in some sense, be psychological. Such discrepancies underscore that making sense of pain is a fragile endeavor, beset by interactional difficulties and ambiguities of meaning. Therefore, while explanatory frames may be potent tools of meaning-making and causal attribution, not all potential meanings will be embraced readily. Some may be perceived as threatening or reproachful, as we will see in the next chapter.

"Sticky" brains came to stand in for a host of relational complexities in the West Clinic's local discourse. Ironically, then, despite the biological reductionism implied by this clinical signifier, caring for a sticky brain meant caring for a family. In the next chapter, I pick up this thread to examine how adolescent chronic pain was always interwoven with ongoing family processes, intimacies, and longer trajectories of care, making it all the more difficult to tease apart cause and effect, both social and embodied.

# 4

# Treating the Family

The family is immediately identified and indicated as, if not
exactly the cause of insanity, at least its occasion.
—Michel Foucault, *Psychiatric Power*

I'd say a really high percentage of them could get better if . . .
their parents would let them.
—Nina Herrera, clinical coordinator, West Clinic

One day, a medical student named Cynthia Marantz presented a challenging case to the pain team in the West Clinic's team meeting. Emilia,
a young woman in her early twenties, had been referred to Dr. Novak
through a friend of a friend. Her chronic pain had begun after a car accident several years earlier, but a complex psychosocial history seemed to
intensify her pain problems and complicate this seemingly straightforward cause. Emilia's parents had divorced when she was quite young,
and she harbored substantial resentment toward her father, while she
described her mother as emotionally unavailable. Now she was depressed
and spent most of her time at home, avoiding social contact. Cynthia and
Dr. Novak indicated that she had appeared anxious and teary-eyed
throughout her visit.

Prior to coming to the West Clinic, Emilia had completed a seven-
week intensive program in an adult pain clinic nearby, which included
aqua-therapy, psychotherapy, and various other therapeutic modalities,
but had seen little relief of her symptoms. In fact, she had developed a
skin reaction to the trigger-point injections that the clinic had prescribed. Dr. Novak knew the psychologist that Emilia had been seeing
as part of the adult pain clinic, and felt that her approach was too psychodynamic. She preferred to see Emilia with someone who could do

cognitive behavioral therapy (CBT) and would teach her concrete coping skills.[1] The only thing that had truly been helping, Emilia maintained, was a retired chiropractor who came to her house several times a week to treat her. Dr. Novak believed that the chiropractor was helping Emilia because he was providing structure—making her walk outside twenty minutes per day—and taking an interest in her well-being. In short, she suggested, he was acting as a substitute father figure, while the psychologist had served as a nurturing maternal type. Both clinicians were compensating for Emilia's unfulfilled family roles.

Dr. Novak's interpretations intrigued me. Although she had disparaged the psychologist's psychodynamic orientation, she offered a classic psychoanalytic reading of the therapeutic enactment of family roles. More strikingly, however, the tone of this explanatory discourse seemed patently different from the neurobiological model of pain that had become so familiar to me on the clinic floor.

In this chapter, I explore how neurobiological and psychodynamic explanatory frames were stitched together over time. I focus especially on the West Clinic's team meetings as a site of negotiation of blame to illustrate the different explanations that took shape in what I have referred to as backstage and onstage clinical spaces. As the sociologist Renee Anspach has observed, "Rarely do doctors directly reveal their assumptions about patients when talking to them; it is in talking and writing to other doctors about patients that cultural assumptions, beliefs, and values are displayed more directly."[2] By opening an analytic space onto what clinicians said about patients behind closed doors, I engage such assumptions, beliefs, and values more explicitly.

As we have already seen, Dr. Novak's clinical explanatory model attributed pain to a flaw in the patient's neurobiological wiring. This model of pain laid the groundwork for a therapeutic approach that emphasized individual responsibility, because intervention was to occur at the level of individual neurobiology. Despite the centrality of this ideology of individual responsibility, however, another prevailing counterlogic circulated throughout the clinic that targeted parents as an important site of intervention and blame.

When I asked Craig Davies, the clinic's cranial sacral therapist, how the West Clinic's patients differed from other patients that he saw in his private practice, he responded: "The first thing that comes to mind is that the pain patients, most of them are, you know, between ten and twenty, that they are the ones whose source of the pain is social or environmental, and that they're trapped. Because they're—they're stuck with families that are, you know, crazy. For lack of a better word." Craig described a particularly poignant case: a patient with chronic abdominal pain who had been emotionally abused by his adoptive mother. It was not until the patient found the emotional strength to express his suffering and resist his mother that his pain went away. This logic figured chronic pain as an intelligible somatic response to psychological trauma, an idea with a strong basis in the clinical literature, stretching back to Freud.[3] In order to overcome the pain, patients had to deal with the psychological stressors that precipitated it, and these stressors were often linked to the family. As one clinician put it succinctly, "Kids are vessels of their families' traumas."[4]

While Craig's description signaled a case of overt abuse, in other cases, more muted forms of familial pathology—such as Emilia's absent mother—though not explicitly abusive, nevertheless exacerbated children's pain or complicated their recovery. For example, after their parents left the room, many patients confessed tearfully that a bout of headaches or stomachaches had started after the parents divorced. "Even if you have pain because you have a brain tumor . . . it's also a good model to try to understand why the pain is as strong as it is," the art therapist Laurel Handelman pointed out. "And often it's, you know, the patient is not cared for properly, or there is a depression which is not cared for, the patient is too much alone or too much *not* alone, or—so it always has a psychosocial implication. Even with pain which we know where it comes from." Laurel's comments underscore the distinction between proximal and distal cause. Even if the pain team truly believed that chronic pain was fundamentally neurobiological, this did not diminish the possibility that some form of psychosocial distress contributed to the illness trajectory.

From a psychodynamic perspective, then, the family was an important site of therapeutic intervention. One of the goals of this chapter is to examine how the discourse of individual responsibility for treatment was complicated by the discourse of family blame, and how these discourses, in turn, were overlaid with different causal attributions and explanatory frames. In doing so, I seek to disrupt the notion of the singular, autonomous patient that has long been so prevalent in Western biomedical settings.

A second, related goal is to illustrate that treatment was aimed, not only at managing pain, but also at prescribing moral ideas about what constitutes good parenting, and, moreover, what constitutes a good family. Here, my concern with "the family" reflects a primary focus on the parent-child relationship, which tends to dominate contemporary middle-class American families.[5] I argue that pediatric pain treatment is a project of socializing patients and their parents into specific moral and cultural worldviews vis-à-vis adolescent development, family roles, and desirable parenting practices. Throughout this process, relationships, caregiving patterns, and the division of household labor all became targets of change, and parents were rendered especially vulnerable to widespread clinical judgment. Thus, "making patients" (and parents) in the clinic was intimately tied to the production of class and gender positions.[6]

In what follows, I first situate this discussion within a broader exploration of cultural conundrums of adolescent autonomy. Then, after briefly introducing the West Clinic's team meetings as a venue for arbitrating competing explanatory frameworks for pain, the remainder of the chapter focuses on a single case in which a patient's family became a key target of blame.

## AMBIVALENT AUTONOMY

On a balmy Mexico morning in March 2010, I sat in a hotel ballroom crowded with physicians, psychologists, and nurses. I was the lone anthropologist interloper, or at least I assumed so, who had come to sunny Acapulco to attend this convention, an international meeting of pediatric pain clinicians and researchers. We were listening to a prominent pediatric pain physician from western Europe give a keynote presentation about multidisciplinary pain treatment. The clinical program he directed was the only tertiary-care center handling pediatric pain in his country, which was not at all small by European standards. The range of clinical services offered was impressive. His team included pediatricians, clinical psychologists, child and adolescent psychiatrists, pediatric nurses, physiotherapists, occupational therapists, and social workers.

When it came time for the question and answer session, a petite woman strode briskly to the aisle, where a microphone had been positioned so that the speaker could take questions from the audience. "And what about the parents?" she asked. I learned later that the woman was a leading pediatric pain physician in a neighboring country.

"We believe parents are very important," the male doctor began confidently. "But we believe more in the power of children than in the power of parents." As the conversation progressed, the female doctor continued to express her skepticism, while the male doctor stood his ground. "It's not proven that you can't treat the family through the child," he said. There was something about the tenor of this exchange that seemed well rehearsed, as if this particular debate had been cycled through before. Their disagreement had the air of a staged clinical performance, with each physician trying to persuade the audience of his or her view of treatment, yet here the audience members were not patients and families but clinical colleagues and researchers.

Later in the week, I found the opportunity to speak with each of them about their respective philosophies of care in the open-air hotel lobby. The male doctor maintained that, because the prospects for changing a family are not very good, it is better to focus treatment on the child. "The chance to really change a family is not very high, we believe," he explained. "So you have to educate, you have to train the child to cope with those things." The female doctor, on the other hand, believed that if the parent does not engage with treatment, it is impossible to move forward with the child. She told me that she and her colleagues feel passionately that parents are essential to treatment, but not everyone does, and she asked whether I had encountered such controversies in my research. I had, as a matter of fact, identified similarly conflicting discourses surrounding the family's role in treatment in my own research in the United States, and I was intrigued to learn that some of the same issues were at stake globally in pediatric pain medicine.

The two physicians' divergent opinions about the role of parents in treatment reflect the difficulty of reconciling an emphasis on adolescent autonomy and responsibility, so prevalent in Western psychology, with an equally prevalent inclination to hold parents responsible for their children's success. While older anthropological theories suggested that societies varied between independent/individualist and interdependent/collectivist orientations that manifested in child-rearing patterns, contemporary accounts recognize that these poles reflect universal tensions rather than discrete types.[7] Such tensions may be selectively mitigated at both individual and cultural levels.[8] For example, the cultural psychologist Annemarie Suizzo suggests that French cultural models of parenting emphasize autonomy *in the service of* affiliation: "Although French mothers stress the importance of developing individual pleasures and qualities, and of being self-assured and autonomous, these goals are justified through the ultimate goal of being able to join groups."[9]

In the West Clinic, in addition to patients' obligation to engage actively in treatment by learning to "rewire" their neurobiological circuitry, clinical socialization included a range of responsibilities for caregivers: ensuring that patients practice their "tools" and "skills" for pain management,[10] implementing a behavioral rewards system to facilitate their return to school and extracurricular activities, and shuttling them back and forth to different therapies (in addition, of course, to paying for them). In each of these tasks, parents were expected to maintain a delicate balance between active involvement in children's treatment and encouraging their self-sufficiency. These incommensurable cultural logics reflect an underlying ambivalence in middle-class American family life that is encapsulated by the sociologist Annette Lareau's notion of concerted cultivation—the idea that parents, paradoxically, encourage their children's independence by actively shaping their strengths and talents.[11]

One problem with such ambivalent expectations for children's dependency, however, is that they set up clinicians to blame parents when children did not get better. Charlotte LeFevre surmised, "The ones that I think have a lower percentage are the ones where there are such huge family issues . . . that they can feel great in this chair and they go out the door and you hear Mom, you know, or Dad or whatever. It's undone as soon as they get out to the sidewalk. And my heart goes out to those kids." Although targeting parents as a direct cause of pain was somewhat rare in the clinic, nearly all of the clinicians on the pain team explicitly recognized the family as a constraint on the recovery process, as well as a supportive resource. Consequently, they went to great lengths to socialize parents regarding pain management strategies.

Dr. Novak handled such discussions delicately and expertly. In one particularly noteworthy case, she began by mentioning to the mother that she was a mother herself, and now a grandmother, so she understood that when your child is suffering, you want to do whatever you can to help get them out of it. "I'm guilty of it too," she acknowledged. The mother admitted, without any prodding, that she was probably overprotective. Then she said, in a very good-natured way, "So you're saying I need treatment, too?" Dr. Novak responded by saying that she thought it could be very helpful to go to a psychologist to help reshape your behavior and interactions. She framed the task as a need to switch paradigms, or belief systems; the psychological treatment would be more of a psycho-educational process. This approach was extremely effective, because Dr. Novak got the mother to arrive at the desired conclusion but let her think that it was her own idea. In the end, the mother responded positively to the idea of psychotherapy and acknowledged that it made a lot of sense to her.

This example highlights the subtle ways in which Dr. Novak worked clinically to redirect parental intrusions and scaffold children's autonomy. At the same time, it also reveals how parental behavior quickly became implicated in children's pain management, as part of a larger project of treating the family. Of course, such tactful framing of inadvertent missteps was particularly useful in onstage clinical interactions. These discussions took a different shape behind the clinic's closed doors.

## THE CLINIC BACKSTAGE

The West Clinic's weekly team meetings were one venue in which I was particularly likely to observe the circulation of more overt discourses of parental blame. Each week, the clinical team gathered for an hour-long meeting. In addition to hearing brief case presentations from Dr. Novak, Dr. Petrosian, and a rotating cast of medical students about the new patients that had come to the clinic that week, team members had the opportunity to raise concerns about specific patients and seek input from the group.

Before each meeting, Nina Herrera, the clinical coordinator, e-mailed the clinicians and asked them to provide names of patients to put on a list for discussion at that week's meeting. A clinician might put a name on the list if she had an upcoming appointment with a new patient and wanted to learn more about the patient from others who had seen her. This enabled clinicians to seek input about treatment plans and specific goals to emphasize. It also permitted them to do a significant amount of their history-taking before ever meeting a patient—a timesaving mechanism that was highly valued by families, who did not usually relish having to tell the same story over and over again to multiple clinicians, particularly when they were paying for the privilege of doing so.

A second group of patients discussed at team meetings included patients whom clinicians viewed as particularly challenging. For such patients, the team meetings presented an unparalleled opportunity to seek feedback from peers about how to handle thorny clinical dilemmas. Here, the multidisciplinary expertise of the clinical team was an important resource for addressing complex problems. The overall spirit of these discussions was egalitarian and participatory. Although Dr. Novak functioned as team "quarterback," as one clinician put it, the pain team was committed to an ethos of collegiality and collaboration, and Dr. Novak eschewed the hierarchical organization common in many clinical settings. Therefore, despite some occasional grumbling about certain clinicians monopolizing the discussion, most regarded the team meetings as a valuable learning experience, through which they continuously expanded their professional knowledge.

The downside of this harmonious atmosphere was that it made clinicians much less likely to express overt disagreement or to question one another's assumptions and judgments. Only one case stands out for inspiring staunch disagreement during the course of my fieldwork. The patient was a seventeen-year-old boy who had been severely injured in a car accident, with his father driving. According to Dr. Petrosian, the patient's mother resented her son because his medical expenses had interfered with her extravagant lifestyle, and the parents were experiencing serious marital problems. Meanwhile, the patient himself had major anger issues and had thrown a vase of his mother's against the wall in a fit of rage. Dr. Novak and Rebecca Hunter had a characteristically psychoanalytic interpretation of this event: the vase was shaped like the mother, thus symbolizing the patient's anger toward her.

Several weeks after the patient was first introduced at a team meeting, a dramatic difference of opinion with regard to the details of the case emerged. At the time, I noted that this type of disagreement was rare in this setting. Dr. Petrosian and Dr. Sterling maintained that the patient's mother was very controlling and emotionally abusive, citing as evidence the fact that she would not let her son get his driver's permit, which he viewed as the only thing that would release him from his depression. Nearly everyone else on the team, however, read the situation very differently. They thought that if there was any danger in the family, it emanated from the father, who had been physically abusive in the past. In contrast, they viewed the mother's behavior as entirely understandable given the history of a traumatic accident. Dr. Novak was very vocal about her different interpretation, which was buttressed in turn by Arlene Weiss, Rebecca Hunter, and Charlotte LeFevre. The gendered nature of this interpretive rift was particularly striking. It was probably not coincidental that Dr. Petrosian and Dr. Sterling had a very different perspective on the case than did Dr. Novak and the rest of the female therapists, who, all mothers themselves, were much more inclined to sympathize with the patient's mother. (Craig Davies, the only other male in the room during this disagreement, was silent for much of the discussion.)

Still, such overt disagreement was rare in my experience. It was far more likely for the clinicians to view the team meetings as a valuable opportunity to coordinate treatment for complex patients, many of whom were being treated by multiple members of the pain team at once. For these patients, regular meetings enabled clinicians to share information and prioritize treatment goals across different therapeutic modalities. For example, if a family determined that they could only afford for their child to see one outside clinician, the team might decide which clinician's services would be most beneficial to the patient.

The meetings also provided an opportunity to work out how clinicians shared and distributed different therapeutic roles. Some patients developed closer relationships with certain clinicians if their personalities clicked. As a result, team members sometimes took on nontraditional roles. For example, early in her treatment, Claire Joffe, the patient whose story I turn to next, came to view Tess Bergman, the yoga instructor, as her primary confidante, while remaining more distant from Laurel Handelman, her individual psychotherapist. Although such situations could provoke some initial awkwardness, the regular contact between team members brought such discomfiture into the open and helped to mitigate hurt feelings.

## THE JOFFE FAMILY

The patient who most captured the attention of the pain team for several months of my fieldwork was a fourteen-year-old girl named Claire Joffe, whom I followed closely over the course of her eight months of treatment in the West Clinic. Like many of the clinic's patients, Claire displayed a mysterious set of symptoms that evaded a clear diagnostic explanation. The initial problem that drove Claire and her parents, Trish and Ricky, to a series of orthopedists, neurologists, and pain specialists before finally landing in the West Clinic was an agonizing pain, stretching from her lower back through her right hip and thigh, that had begun following a basketball injury. Yet it was a set of related, distressing symptoms that emerged much later that forced her to withdraw from school and to enter a home-schooling program for the duration of her ninth-grade year.

Several weeks before her first visit to the clinic, in March 2009, Claire began to experience a series of panic attacks that appeared as seizure-like episodes where her body shook uncontrollably. She also began to pass out up to twenty times per day, and she sometimes fell and hurt herself as she was losing consciousness. After several weeks, around the time of her first West Clinic appointment, the panic attacks progressed into night terrors, where Claire would, without awakening, stir from a prone position, rise, and thrash around violently, kicking and pushing her parents if they tried to restrain her. The episodes could last for fifteen or twenty minutes at a time, several times per night.

Ricky recorded several of these incidents on his home camcorder. Although to many of the clinicians it seemed somewhat perverse for him to have filmed his daughter at the height of her vulnerability, I later came to believe that he did so because he doubted that anyone would otherwise believe his account. The episodes were disturbing to watch. There was considerable struggling and wrestling while Trish and Ricky attempted to restrain Claire, and occasionally, she would escape her parents' grasp and injure herself. Ricky and Trish were quite concerned that Claire would hurt herself seriously during these episodes. She often arched her neck backward, and they worried that it might snap. Ricky, a freelance designer who worked from home, maintained that someone needed to be close to Claire twenty-four hours a day, and since Trish worked for an architectural firm, he took on this role himself.

Claire began seeing Dr. Sterling a few weeks before her first appointment with Dr. Novak, because he had an opening in his schedule sooner, and Dr. Novak thought that he could help treat her psychiatric symptoms. By the time she arrived at the West Clinic, Claire had tried numerous medications, including Neurontin, Elavil, and Vicodin for pain; Ativan and clonazepam (both benzodiazepines) for anxiety; and Zoloft (an SSRI), which targeted both pain and anxiety. On at least one occasion, the Joffes had dialed 911 because they were so worried by Claire's seizures and panic attacks. She had undergone neurological testing after visiting an emergency room, but it did not uncover a physiological cause. When not having an active panic episode, Claire was extremely lethargic and withdrawn, but her complex pharmaceutical profile made it difficult to sort out symptoms from side effects.

The family was quickly absorbed into the clinic's therapeutic fold. During my fieldwork, no other family participated in the West Clinic's therapies to the extent that the Joffe family did, and because their insurance company did not cover many of the team's services, they did so under considerable financial duress, spending more than $700 per week at the height of Claire's treatment. I offer the following vignettes to illustrate how the pain team applied different explanatory frames over time, shifting from the neurobiological explanation of Claire's symptoms employed in the clinic intake appointments to a more psychodynamic orientation. In doing so, I demonstrate how, in this clinical milieu, treatment not only entailed treating an individual patient, but also treating a family.

The discussion that follows is organized in terms of three explanatory frameworks for Claire's symptoms: neurobiology, trauma and repression, and social roles in the family. However, it is important to emphasize that these explanatory frames were not applied in successive, linear fashion. I have been confronted with a representational challenge in conveying the ambivalence with which the pain team approached Claire's case, sometimes employing overlapping explanatory frames and circling back to previously discarded causal attributions. In addressing this task, I was greatly inspired by the anthropologist Sarah Pinto's observation that the anthropologist, as analyst, encounters challenges in framing a case that in some respects mirror the interpretive demands of clinical work.[12] Nuanced anthropological case studies uphold the multilayered contingent meanings of clinical histories and illustrate how competing, even incommensurable, narrative threads offer different implications for where we locate the cause of suffering. Therefore, the illusion of order imposed by the framing that follows should not entirely efface the overwhelming sense of uncertainty that Claire's case provoked.

*Neurobiology*

Like most of Dr. Novak's patients, Claire fit the profile of the prototypical West Clinic patient. She was a strong student, and despite some unevenness in her performance, had tested at the high end of the gifted scale. She was also talented in both athletics and the arts, an unusual combination in the clinic. At my first meeting with the Joffes, Trish and Ricky showed me sketchbooks filled with exquisite pencil drawings and pointed out a series of sculptures displayed prominently on their living-room bookshelf that easily might have been made by a professional artist. It was clearly sports, however, that occupied center stage in family life. Both Claire and her eleven-year-old sister Vanessa played on multiple teams, and prior to her injury, Claire's participation on softball, basketball, and soccer teams had been a key part of her identity. She had even played on a boys' Little League team from the age of four, which set her apart from the many young athletes that I met through my work in the West Clinic. Ricky, who had worked as a photographer, proudly showed me shots of Claire on the baseball field that he had taken when she was a young girl.

At their first visit to the West Clinic, the Joffes received a generic explanation of Claire's troubles that framed both her pain and her psychiatric symptoms as neurobiological. After learning about Claire's background, Dr. Novak repeated what had become, for me, a familiar refrain: "We tend to call our clinic the smart clinic because there's something about the neurobiology of being really smart [which leads to chronic pain]." Dr. Novak assured the Joffes that she was not mystified by Claire's story—she had seen many creative, athletic patients just like Claire, with similar stories to tell. She diagnosed Claire with myofascial pain: pain that results from tender points in the muscle tissue that activate the nerve-signaling system and "turn on" neural networks, creating hypersensitive areas. She also indicated that Claire's panic-like episodes were likely pseudo-seizures, rather than manifestations of a true seizure disorder. This was not to say that her symptoms were fabricated, but rather that they resulted from an excess of neural activity.

Here again, Dr. Novak's explanatory rhetoric tied Claire's symptoms to her personal attributes: it was because she was smart and creative that her nervous system had become overstimulated. As Dr. Novak explained, "Now that you have a pain problem . . . your attention is being focused. Because you're good at noticing thi- I mean, a writer, an artist is very observant. So you're also observant of your own inner signaling. And so your attention goes to those different changes in your body and then that gets your—what's called your sympathetic nervous system, your fight or flight [reflex], you know, the part of you that makes more adrenaline and makes your heart beat faster and makes you have hot and cold flashes and makes you dizzy. That gets turned on." Using this logic, Dr. Novak drew a clear causal link from Claire's smartness and creativity to a hypervigilance toward bodily changes, to an activated sympathetic nervous system, and finally to the seizures: "And when all of this is going on, it keeps things in. And that's sort of a formula for the pseudo-seizures. . . . It's the body's safety valve." The metaphor of a safety valve suggested that the pseudo-seizures offered a mechanical function: to release pent-up neurosensory activity and restore Claire's sympathetic nervous system to its normal functioning.

Dr. Novak recommended that Claire stop taking Neurontin, because her pain was not neuropathic, and it was probably making her feel "drugged out and tired." She also eliminated the Elavil, because of two abnormal electrocardiograms that she reviewed in the chart room during a break.[13] Dr. Novak explained that her goal was to stabilize Claire's anxiety so that she could work on other therapies long-term. Claire could stay on Ativan and clonazepam for now, but Dr. Novak's goal was to eliminate them; she recommended Lexapro instead, because of its low side effects. She also mentioned that she had discussed this plan with Dr. Sterling when she went into the chart room. In addition to the pills, Dr. Novak wrote a prescription for Lidoderm, an anesthetic lidocaine patch that Claire could apply to the site of her pain.

Just as she had with Michael Harris, Dr. Novak emphasized that Claire's intelligence would be an important therapeutic asset. "So if we looked at an electrical engineer looking at the wiring we'd see a turned on system," she said. "And that's not uncommon but it tends to happen more in kids who are smart. So that's the downside about being smart. The good side is that, that it will also help you use your smartness to undo that." Dr. Novak made several referrals to clinicians on the pain team: Laurel Handelman for art therapy, to provide an alternative "release mechanism" for Claire's anxiety; Charlotte LeFevre for hypnotherapy, "to start changing those pain circuits in creative ways"; and Tess Bergman for Iyengar yoga, to work to restore Claire's muscular functioning and prevent her hypermobility from causing further injuries. "We all work as a team," Dr. Novak explained. "I'll be letting them know about you. They'll be working in their area of expertise with you, but we'll all be communicating as a team."

*Trauma and Repression*

The following week, the pain team sat around the conference table, talking about Claire. By this point, she had had appointments with Tess, Laurel, and Charlotte, all of whom were rankled by Ricky's behavior and what they perceived as his overly protective stance toward his daughter. Ricky had hovered close to Claire at her appointments, afraid that she might lose consciousness and fall. That this did not occur in their presence made them all the more suspicious that his close attention was unwarranted. Laurel, in particular, was perturbed by an image from Claire's sketchbook that suggested the possibility of a conflict with her father.

It was not particularly unusual for the pain team to view clinic parents as intrusive or overprotective. What began to set Claire's case apart, however, was a report from Craig Davies that raised the possibility of a prior trauma. Although Craig had not been on Dr. Novak's original list of referrals, she had mentioned toward the end of Claire's first appointment that massage could be very helpful for myofascial pain, and that the clinic had a wonderful craniosacral therapist who could come to a patient's home and do a massage. The Joffes had called

Craig the previous night, and he had offered to come to their house around bedtime, in the hope that a calming massage might help Claire have a night of uninterrupted sleep. The plan had worked, and she had slept soundly from 8 P.M. to 6:30 the next morning.

Craig appeared troubled in recounting his session with Claire. He described how the Joffes had set up mattresses on the floor in the living room so that Ricky and Trish could sleep on either side of her and guard her if she got up during the night during one of her night terrors. They had also played some of the disturbing video footage of one of Claire's nighttime episodes for him. During the massage, he recalled, she had acted "like a sponge for safe, nurturing, I think male, touch." Her pelvis and chest seemed very "locked down," meaning rigid, and at one point she had had an intense coughing spell.

Craig's account raised incongruous signs, which the pain team struggled to interpret. Both the coughing and the "locked-down" chest and pelvis had been understood in prior team meetings as indices of prior abuse or trauma.[14] At the same time, Rebecca Hunter ventured that based on the fact that Claire relaxed so easily with Craig, she doubted that there was a history of abuse, and guessed that it might be a boundary issue instead, which the family's sleeping arrangements and Claire's lack of privacy only seemed to confirm. Without reaching any firm conclusions, there was a strong consensus around the table of the need to work with the family. At Dr. Novak's suggestion, Arlene Weiss, one of the clinic's psychologists, agreed to meet with the Joffes if they were willing.

Already at this early point in her therapeutic trajectory, Claire's symptoms had taken on a second layer of meaning. Although she undoubtedly fit the profile of the clinic's prototypical patient, and Dr. Novak had assured Claire that her pain and pseudo-seizures were related to her "smart" and "creative" neurons, the conversation around the table belied the straightforward logic of the neurobiological frame. Instead, the clinicians examined brief encounters to mine them for underlying clues about how an unknown prior trauma might be contributing to Claire's symptomatology. In this way, a fleeting comment or gesture could be read and reread by the pain team to help make Claire's experience legible.

At Claire's third clinic visit, two weeks later, I observed a subtle shift in Dr. Novak's explanatory stance with the Joffes. The previous week, Dr. Novak had arranged a hospital admission to monitor Claire's neurological activity overnight, and, as she had suspected, the EEG revealed only normal brain activity. Toward the end of the appointment, Dr. Novak summarized where they were with Claire's treatment: "Whatever the behavioral stuff, I truly believe you have pain and we're gonna work on the pain. Everything else that we're talking about . . . doesn't negate the fact that you really have pain." At this point, Claire, who was already lying down on the examination table, lost consciousness, and Dr. Novak continued to address her parents, patting Claire's leg while talking. "And then the behavioral part is what we really need—it's almost like there's a circuit in her brain that's gone into a pattern that when whatever's going on, she's having these dissociative, tune-out reactions. And I think it's unconscious, it's not like she's malingering. It's not like she's doing this purposefully."

To this point, Dr. Novak's explanation was very much aligned with her prior account of the pseudo-seizures. At the first visit, she had suggested that the dissociative episodes resulted from an overstimulated sympathetic nervous system. However, she had also drawn a causal link between the pain and the seizures, proposing that Claire's hypervigilance to her pain had activated her sympathetic nervous system and set off the behavioral response. Dr. Novak now understood this relationship quite differently. "I think there is something going on that we don't know about that has triggered these behaviors," she explained to the Joffes. "I don't know if it's an incident that happened at school that nobody knows about. I mean, something has set off these—and it's not just the pain. I mean, the pain is there, we'll address the pain, but it's not that the pain is so bad it's causing this. There is something else that's creating so much stress internally that it's adding to the pain and also triggering these behaviors. And I think that's why the work with Dr. [Laurel] Handelman is gonna be important." The critical point here, of course, is: *it's not that the pain is . . . causing this.* This assessment points to a psychological cause that predated the pain altogether. Thus, rather than attributing Claire's symptoms solely to a problem of neurobiological wiring, Dr. Novak complicated her prior diagnostic narrative by suggesting that a traumatic event or repressed memory was contributing to Claire's distress.

Psychological models of trauma and dissociation, on the one hand, and neurobiological models of seizure activity, on the other, locate the cause of suffering differently. In the former case, the cause is external to the individual but produces intrapsychic effects. In the neurological model, however, both cause and effect are contained within an individual body.[15] Moreover, whether we locate Claire's suffering in her neurobiology or in psychological trauma has important consequences for the moral stance from which her behavior is viewed. If Claire's dissociative episodes result from a neurobiological problem, the cause lies beyond her control. Yet if, instead, the dissociative episodes result from a traumatic event, an external agent might be to blame. At the same time, insofar as the proximal cause of the seizures would point to a failure of psychic integration, personal responsibility would also be less easily evaded.

Before leaving the clinic that day, Ricky reminded Claire of a question that had been troubling her: *Am I crazy?* Ricky recalled how a hospital neurologist had dodged the question by asking, "What is crazy?" Dr. Novak reiterated that she thought that there was something neuromuscular that was causing the pain. But she also thought that there was something else, something "eating you inside in terms of stress," something that Claire was not remembering. When Claire interjected that she honestly could not think of anything that could have happened, Dr. Novak responded: "Yeah, I totally understand. And it may be there's not. I mean, if you could remember it, you would say it, and your body wouldn't keep reacting." Dr. Novak compared Claire to "a little volcano that periodically erupts," assuring her that they would work with Laurel to get some of her stress out through creative means so that it would not continue to build up. "So I don't know if that's an answer," Dr. Novak summed up. "But I don't think you're crazy."

After several weeks, the violent nighttime episodes diminished. In their place, however, a new behavior emerged during Claire's dissociative states: she unconsciously began signing "S-I-M-P-L-E-L-I-F-E-N-O-P-A-I-N" in American Sign Language (ASL), which she had taken classes in. Ricky showed me several recordings he had made on his home camcorder of Claire in this state. In the first, Claire sat up straight with her head hung low, hair in front of her face, and arms stretched out to either side of her body. She signed with both hands in a graceful, rhythmic fashion, almost as if she were dancing. With each hand, she made the same gesture, using a sweeping movement between letter forms to denote breaks. Then, after several seconds of signing, she slumped over and Trish caught her and laid her down. In the second series, Claire was lying down on her stomach with her arms stretched out in front of her. At one point, her body began to shake gently, which I recognized as the mark of the pseudo-seizure, but she lay peacefully asleep for the rest of the time.

Around this time, Laurel brought in some of Claire's artwork to one of the team meetings and highlighted a drawing of a hand making a peace sign. Laurel had asked Claire to talk about the drawing, and Claire had said that it meant "surrender." Laurel interpreted this as Claire surrendering to her symptoms. She contrasted this image with a picture of a clenched fist that Claire had drawn at an earlier session. The picture represented a dream that Claire had had about a time when she had received a trophy for being the only girl on a boy's Little League team. Claire had described this time as the height of her confidence. The fist was clenched because she was tired of having lost it all; she was tired of being dependent.

If the peace sign represented Claire's acceptance of loss and dependence, then her cryptic message in ASL might likewise be seen as the vital enactment of her surrender. In both scenes, the hands figured centrally, conveying the body's defeat. For an artist and athlete, the significance of the hands was their centrality to her self-reliance. That they were communicating an urgent message to her unconscious self suggested a pathway to healing.

And yet, while Laurel's reading suggested therapeutic progress, Trish and Ricky remained shaken up. They indicated that Claire's signing was by far the scariest element of her unconscious repertoire, and described her behavior as like something out of the movie *The Exorcist*. Their fearful reaction derived in part from their inability to decipher the meaning of Claire's insistent messages, due to their unfamiliarity with ASL. While Claire's violent, aggressive episodes were undeniably frightening, the specificity of her signed accounts suggested a pressing communication from a source, if not external to Claire, then at least deeply submerged in her subconscious. Thus, Trish and Ricky continued to worry, hoping that Claire's continued treatment would offer further interpretive clues.

### Social Roles in the Family

In the following weeks, the pain team gradually abandoned their suspicions of trauma, becoming more and more convinced that the family's sleeping arrangements and Ricky's close surveillance were perpetuating Claire's distress. With Trish working outside the home, Ricky had taken on much of the responsibility for Claire's care, spending his days with her at home and driving her to almost daily therapy appointments with members of the pain team. He was reluctant to leave Claire alone for her sessions with Charlotte, Laurel, and Tess, even though she had never passed out during these sessions, a fact they interpreted as evidence that her loss of consciousness was somehow related to Ricky's control. Ricky had also gotten into the habit of taking Claire to the bathroom, because she had passed out while sitting on the toilet, which the team, relying on implicit norms mandating privacy between family members of different sexes, deemed inappropriate behavior for the father of an adolescent female.

At an early meeting, Laurel offered a tentative analysis: Ricky, as an out-of-work freelancer, had nothing to do, and lived vicariously through his daughter's talents. The team came to suspect that Claire was unconsciously reacting to her father's control and all-consuming attention by periodically losing consciousness, and that her dissociative episodes would not subside until she regained her independence. They viewed Ricky as overly enmeshed in his daughter's life, while they perceived soft-spoken Trish as timid, cowering to Ricky's authority. The general consensus was that Claire needed to spend more time with Trish and less with Ricky.

In clinic visits with the Joffes, Dr. Novak stated the importance of Claire returning to her bedroom, subtly at first, and then more emphatically. When, during one April clinic visit, Ricky explained that Claire needed to clean up her bedroom first, Dr. Novak looked at Claire and said, firmly, "You're going to do that today. And sleep in your own room tonight." Dr. Novak instructed the Joffes to put pillows around Claire's bed to protect her in case she fell during a nighttime dissociative episode. At the team meeting two days later, Dr. Novak read aloud snippets of an e-mail from Ricky reporting that Claire had finally gotten her room ready to move back in. Dr. Novak editorialized as she read, "See, she was just wanting to have some limits set." Claire had made her own breakfast and gone to the bathroom on her own. Ricky had added, with his characteristic dry wit, "I handed her the want ads and told her to go get a job."

Although the group's stance toward Ricky seemed considerably more positive than it had been a few weeks earlier, there were still many problems. Arlene Weiss reported that Ricky dominated the couple's therapy sessions, frequently interrupting his wife, so that Arlene had to actively intervene to facilitate Trish's participation. Charlotte asked Arlene whether she had a sense of what the relationship between Claire and Trish was like, intuiting that this would be key, but Arlene had limited insight into it. Meanwhile, Craig had observed in the Joffes' home that Trish was beginning to assert herself more in front of Ricky. He also sensed that Trish believed that Claire was beginning to get better due to the time that she and Trish spent together.

Part of the problem, Arlene explained, was that Trish was working two jobs. Dr. Novak chimed in, "We need to get him working as well. *He* needs to be combing the want ads!" Dr. Novak suggested that Arlene structure a "behavioral plan" with the objective of adjusting parental roles.[16] Charlotte worried about offending Ricky. If he thought they identified him as the problem, he might take his anger out on Trish, and if anger in the household escalated, Claire would remain "stuck." Craig drew on Chinese philosophy to suggest: "Can you frame it like yin and yang? Like she needs the balance of male and female."

At the same meeting, someone mentioned that Claire's younger sister, Vanessa, was going to visit a family friend out of town who did not have children her age, and that Claire might likewise be going to visit friends of the Joffes who did not have children. The team thought that this pattern was strange and wondered whether Claire might have been subject to some abuse by one of these family friends. Might it be possible that Ricky suspected that something like this had occurred, and that his protective behavior was a reaction to these suspicions? Here, competing interpretive threads were woven together, with the team circling back to the question of abuse, even as they appeared to blame the Joffes for what they viewed as questionable parental judgment.

The conversation had begun to take on the air of a mystery novel, with everyone working to fit together the pieces of a puzzle whose overall landscape had not yet taken shape. Cheryl Mattingly has written that the detective story is a canonical genre of clinical work. "The clinician as sleuth has the task of investigating medical mysteries," she suggests, "identifying the (hidden) criminal who perpetrates crimes inside a patient's body, leaving traces in the form of symptoms and signs that present puzzles to be deciphered."[17] In Claire's case, however, the hidden offender was less an elusive disease than a compelling semiotic framework linking symptoms with cause. However eager the team seemed to be to discount a history of abuse, they were nevertheless unprepared to reject this possibility entirely. What troubled them most was a sense that something as yet unknown might hold the key to Claire's distress.

Hovering over this clinical detective work was the haunting presence of the law.[18] The possibility of trauma exposed Claire's distress to legal as well as clinical action, with disturbing implications for the family. The possibility of abuse acted simultaneously as a clinical sign, diagnosing Claire's symptoms; a moral sign, explaining unnatural intimacies; and a persecutory sign, demanding intervention. As in many pediatric settings, the pain team was cautious about reporting suspected child abuse to California's Child Protective Services. The high standards of evidence required for legal action pose a significant threat that children will experience negative repercussions if a case is reported only to ultimately be dismissed. During the course of my research, the team deliberated over several cases but never, to my knowledge, reported them. Nevertheless, the possibility remained that enough evidence would be uncovered that Claire's case would need to be reported, potentially damaging both the team's relationship with the Joffes and Claire's therapeutic progress. Underlying this backstage detective work was thus a clinical, moral, and also legal responsibility to intervene if abuse was indeed happening.

. . .

It took about six weeks for Dr. Novak to stabilize Claire's pharmaceutical regimen. She had tried Lyrica for a week, but it made her dizzy and disrupted her vision. Although Claire had been quite docile in her first few weekly appointments with Dr. Novak, following the Lyrica, she resolved to be more candid, explaining to me via text message: "I just really haven't been feeling well . . . Trust me. U will here [sic] all about it tomorrow!!! I am going to be very verbal tomorrow with dr. Novak!!! Ur gonna be shocked becuz I am very upset!" The next day in clinic, she announced, "I'm gonna talk. The medication you put me on has not been working. It's made my life a lot worse." If Claire had needed to pluck up her courage to deliver this message, she need not have worried. Dr. Novak apologized for Claire's bad week immediately and told her that she should stop taking Lyrica.

Once Claire was down to taking only Lexapro, she seemed to do much better. Trish attributed this improvement both to Claire's therapeutic work with the pain team and to discontinuing the other medications, which had made her very lethargic. Three weeks after she stopped taking Lyrica, Ricky asked whether Claire would need to continue with the Lexapro. Dr. Novak said she would. When Claire asked what Lexapro did, Dr. Novak said that it "helps to rebalance your system," a euphemistic explanation that made me wonder whether Claire knew that it was an antidepressant.

During the same appointment, Dr. Novak asked to see Claire and her parents separately. First, she spoke with Claire alone and asked how things were going. Now emboldened to speak her mind, Claire said she did not think it was helpful for her to go on seeing the physical therapist, Meg Pratt (who was not one of Dr. Novak's original referrals, but whom she had seen several times), or the psychologist Arlene Weiss, whom she met with in family sessions with her parents. Dr. Novak quickly released Claire from both of these obligations, noting that she already had a lot of appointments. The conversation turned next to family matters. "Have you had more alone time with your mom?" Dr. Novak asked. Claire said that she had had a little, but would like more. "Last week she asked me to do her nails, hair, and makeup," Claire recalled. "We don't do that a lot." They spoke a little about school, and her thoughts about returning. It was April, and Claire was not eager to return before the end of the year, hoping instead for a fresh start in August.

When Trish and Ricky were called back in to the room, Claire told them, "I don't have to go to Dr. Weiss anymore. You do, though!" Ricky turned to Dr. Novak. "We had a question about if we really need to go there." Dr. Novak seized this opportunity to segue into a private conversation with Trish and Ricky. After Claire left the room, Dr. Novak explained that she felt that continued work with Arlene would be a good opportunity for "rebalancing in the family." She broached the family's division of labor cautiously. "And you've been sort of the main one sort of monitoring," she said to Ricky. "And, you know, especially while you're out," she gestured toward Trish. "And . . . with all of those behaviors, it makes you have to monitor even more closely. And I think in a— in a paradoxical way, I think Claire needs you to monitor her less."

She then pushed more explicitly to realign the family system with normative gender roles for middle-class American family life. By this point, Claire's dissociative episodes had substantially improved, and the Joffes were beginning to wonder why they still needed to be in couples therapy if Claire was doing better. Dr. Novak framed it as a preventive effort, to keep Claire from relapsing. She explained very delicately that nothing was broken, but that this was an opportunity for some fine-tuning and rebalancing of family roles, which would be useful with two daughters entering adolescence:

> So it's not that you have to fix a bad relationship. It's not that at all. It's . . . beginning to use their adolescence as sort of a period of reorganizing family systems or the family dynamics just a little bit. It's that tweak during adolescence, especially having two daughters, where, at this point, you know, unless you [gesturing at Ricky] don a wig and change your habitus, you know, daughters need a little more time with their mom. And not that the nurturing and all the other stuff that they're getting from you certainly isn't valuable, and it doesn't mean they shouldn't have time with you, but it—it's those subtle, ah, you know, how do you learn how to be a woman? Well, you learn how to be a woman as a kid from your mother.

Through comments such as these, Dr. Novak worked to socialize a particular cultural model of adolescence in which girls should increasingly spend more time with their mothers so that they could learn to adopt gendered habits, bodily comportment, and normative social roles.

Yet the team's backstage concerns about Ricky supervising Claire in the bathroom suggest that something more than the failure of gendered expectations might be at stake. Dr. Novak's comments to the Joffes exposed as much as they veiled a haunting fear of perversity and unnatural intimacies between kin. Beyond just promoting a specific model of middle-class American family life, the nature and boundaries of Ricky's relationship with his adolescent daughter came under clinical and moral scrutiny.

Such concerns reveal an effort to rehabilitate the family in ways that, on the surface, did not always track with the original impetus for treatment, yet nevertheless seemed important—from the pain team's perspective—to familial ecologies of care. Throughout this discussion, Dr. Novak took great care to avoid a discourse of blame. She even remarked that her own husband had suffered a similar fate when her daughters entered adolescence. Yet while Trish and Ricky received this feedback with striking composure, I often wondered whether other families would withstand a similar level of critical appraisal.

It was at this same appointment that Dr. Novak first acknowledged to the Joffes that she had been exploring the possibility of trauma. "There's still something going on inside," Dr. Novak explained. "You know, I will say that when I've seen kids that have had these major dissociative reactions . . . the first thing as a clinician that I have to think is, is there any kind of abuse, sexual abuse that has happened." She assured Trish and Ricky that she had been feeling less and less concerned about this possibility over time, yet she mentioned that Claire's coughing fits during massage sessions with Craig represented a lingering puzzle:

> So, you know, I have to tell you, that made me think back again to—did she have some experience? And this is all hypothesis based on types of symptoms and past experience. So then there's part of me that's concerned, okay, did something happen at school or somewhere else? Or it could be just whatever emotions. I mean, this is sort of the way the body works, it's like that's the last expulsion, and it may have absolutely nothing to do with anything sexual at all. So, you know, this is the thinking from clinical experience, seeing kids over time. But it makes me feel like there's still a little work to do to get her really stabilized, get whatever is to finish coming out.

Ricky admitted that he had considered these possibilities as well, but he was firmly convinced that there had been no opportunity for something like this to occur, outside of school. "I mean, she barely goes to the mall," he explained. "And between school and soccer practice, that was 100 percent of her time." As for the coughing, he noted that whenever he had an upset stomach, it made him cough. "It could be as simple as she got that from me." When Trish wondered aloud whether it might be related to Claire's asthma, Dr. Novak responded: "You know, it could be any and all of that. It could be that she gets reflux. . . . I was, I guess, being open in terms of what goes on, like all the different possibilities. And the reality is we'll all know in time, or we won't know, but things will just keep improving. And then it won't matter. 'Cause if it's something really bad it'll come out."

· · ·

Slowly, reports of the Joffes' adjustment of the household division of labor trickled in. Claire was becoming more active again, and she and Trish had kicked around a soccer ball in the backyard. Laurel reported a striking difference in Claire's demeanor: the color was back in her face, and she seemed happy. But when Ricky left town on two work-related trips in quick succession in the middle of May, leaving Trish to contend with the domestic responsibilities, I realized that although his departure granted Trish the time alone with her daughters that the team had pushed for, it also put a great deal of pressure on her, as she struggled to balance Claire's intensive therapeutic needs with her already busy schedule.

The team also expressed disapproval of Trish and Ricky's parenting in subtle other ways. Charlotte was taken aback by the fact that when Claire was sick with the flu and needed to cancel an appointment, Claire had been the one to telephone her, rather than Ricky. Likewise, Claire had called her pediatrician's office when some antibiotics she was given caused her to vomit. "She took that on," Charlotte told me. Tess reported to the team that Claire had been very excited about Tess meeting her mother for the first time. Ricky had been out of town on this occasion, and when Trish was late to pick her up, Claire remarked that she was never on time. Tess took this as a small sign that "nobody's taking care of Claire." This seemed a harsh conclusion, given the hectic pace of life (and busy traffic) in the area. Laurel, too, criticized Ricky for driving through the night with Claire on a road trip to visit friends out of state, which Claire had long been promised. Meanwhile, the team provided parenting where they felt that Trish and Ricky were lacking. When Tess helped Claire respond to an older teenage boy who had made sexual overtures via text message, Dr. Novak told the team that Tess had played a "structured parenting role," because Claire was not getting that at home.[19]

I do not have a very good sense of whether (and how) Trish and Ricky experienced such judgments. While my ethnographic alignments were split between the West Clinic team and the family, I developed a much closer relationship with Claire than with either of her parents. While they were certainly cordial to me when I saw them in the clinic, they nevertheless remained somewhat aloof about how Claire's treatment affected them. Moreover, while they quite generously permitted me to intrude into Claire's clinical treatment, they declined my request to videotape in their home.[20]

From Arlene Weiss's reports at team meetings, I do know that Trish and Ricky felt judged on some level. Arlene indicated that the Joffes were unusually embarrassed about some of their family habits that seemed (to me) pretty innocuous, such as watching television during dinner. This may have explained their reluctance to let me film. Arlene also intimated that Trish preferred that certain things not be shared with the team. Yet given the intense level of clinical scrutiny that families expose themselves to by engaging in this sort of treatment, this guardedness is not surprising; in fact, had they not been completely desperate, the Joffes might not have agreed to participate in therapy at all. The couples sessions with Arlene Weiss were the one aspect of Claire's treatment plan to which the Joffes expressed resistance, given the financial burdens of the therapy, and the fact that, in their view, it helped Claire only tangentially. Yet when Dr. Novak stressed its importance, they continued to attend dutifully despite the financial strain.

## BLAMING THE FAMILY IN PEDIATRIC MEDICINE

Claire's symptoms steadily improved during her first four months of treatment. She connected particularly well with Charlotte and Tess, who gave her practical skills, like meditation, yoga poses, and relaxation exercises, which Trish described as "tools for life." Gradually, the dissociative episodes dissipated, and the pain, while still present, became more manageable. Claire slowly resumed her physical activity, taking long walks around her neighborhood with Trish and their dogs. That summer, however, Claire suffered a significant setback when Trish was diagnosed with a serious medical condition and had to undergo surgery quite suddenly. Initially, Claire responded with an increase in night terrors, but they subsided after it became clear that Trish would recover. Although the discourse of family blame eventually lifted, the pain team's failure to pinpoint a concrete physiological cause—and its implicit suggestions about a hidden trauma—indelibly altered Claire's understanding of her condition. Thus, although her pain had improved dramatically, she still felt far from normal.

Claire's story offers no tidy resolution. When I returned to California for a visit during her senior year of high school, I was pleased to see her thriving and more or less pain-free. We spoke of college applications, her new boyfriend, and her excitement over a possible move to a different part of the country. However, we never uncovered the reason for the mysterious symptoms that had plagued her for half of her freshman year, nor did we fully understand how or why they disappeared, although Claire and her family credited the West Clinic fully for her recovery.

The explanatory frameworks outlined here—neurobiology, trauma and repression, and social roles in the family—offer three interpretive schemas for making sense of Claire's illness history. That Claire's dissociative states became less frequent after the Joffes implemented clinical guidelines for restructuring family roles reaffirmed the validity of this explanation to the pain team—though of course it would be difficult to know for sure why this behavior dissipated. Yet hierarchies of causal explanations may offer a false sense of clarity.[21] In this case, they may minimize the lingering ambivalence and recursive reasoning with which we often make sense of suffering.

Avoiding blaming parents in the early phases of treatment serves an important clinical function—namely, affirming the legitimacy of the patient's (and family's) claims and securing therapeutic buy-in. At one conference I attended, an audience member asked a well-known American pediatric pain psychologist about the role of family therapy. He responded that this must be approached delicately, because families do not want to see the child's pain as a psychological problem. Although he did not say so, it also seems quite likely that some parents would experience recommendation of family therapy as an allegation of parental shortcomings. "If you go there too early, you can blow it," he warned.

What nevertheless seems clear is that the onstage diagnostic narrative offered by Dr. Novak's clinical explanatory model—that pain was caused by "smart neurons"—was insufficient for fully interpreting the underlying source of at least some patients' symptoms. Although I have focused here on Claire's story, there were numerous other examples of patients whose pain the team believed to be exacerbated by familial distress. It is therefore important to distinguish between psychodynamic *causes* of pain and factors that interfere with recovery. Regardless of whether a biological cause could be identified, the pain team believed that many families did things, however unwittingly, to perpetuate or exacerbate symptoms.

The most frequently cited example involved parents who asked their children how they were feeling, and in doing so, drew attention to the pain, making it more difficult for the children to distract themselves. At one clinic visit, Jon Morgan, the father of eleven-year-old Zack, told me that Rebecca Hunter wanted them to ignore Zack's pain and screaming. Jon said, "We tried to be supportive but we were told by Rebecca, don't even focus on the pain, don't say you're going to get better. Don't say how are you. Which is kind of counterintuitive." It was obvious from the time I spent with the family that they struggled to put this advice into practice. Every time Zack screamed, the whole family—including Zack's twenty-one-year-old sister—pleaded with him to stop, and Sherri, Zack's mother, repeatedly rubbed his back. Later, Jon told Dr. Novak that that he kept getting into trouble with Rebecca, but that he "felt like a creep" when he didn't respond to Zack's screams.

A less common example, but one that still arose with some regularity, involved parents who were believed to be benefiting from some form of secondary gain as a result of the child's illness. Arlene Weiss explained, "I've seen others where the parents themselves, either because they're having marital problems or don't have a big social circle themselves, sort of glom onto their kids' problem and make it their own in a certain way. So where I said it's symbiotic, it serves a purpose for Mom as well as, let's say, a child who's more dependent."

As such observations make clear, parents make themselves vulnerable by engaging in this kind of biopsychosocial treatment. Sarah Pinto has illustrated that clinical ethics are intimately tied to kin ethics, with clinical rationality deployed, in the case of Indian psychiatry that Pinto considers, to "police the moral boundaries of marriage . . . crafting better, more ideal, mothers, daughters, wives, families, and marriages."[22] In the West Clinic, too, treatment logics were riddled with normative assumptions about gender socialization, intimacy, and the micro-politics of family life. Such accounts of clinical judgment destabilize conventional biomedical notions of the singular, autonomous patient by focusing medicine's normalizing gaze squarely on the family.

Making judgments about parents is a routine feature of pediatric work both in the United States and elsewhere.[23] For Trish and Ricky

Joffe, what was at stake was the insidious way in which putative expert knowledge linked their daughter's suffering to their own parenting. Claims such as Dr. Novak's assertion that "daughters need a little more time with their mom" reflect stocks of cultural knowledge regarding adolescent development and gender norms, revealing sensibilities about care that stretch well beyond the delimited sphere of pain medicine. They also reveal a blurring between exercising clinical judgment and disciplining the family, inasmuch as Dr. Novak admitted to the Joffes that the family roles and division of labor might not be directly related to Claire's pain. Yet more than disciplining gender roles, the pain team's aversion toward Ricky's behavior also revealed a fear of perverse forms of familial intimacy, the threat of which appeared morally questionable to the clinicians. In this way, the clinic came to prescribe, not only treatment for pain, but also a specific vision of what middle-class American family life should be like.

Over the course of Claire's treatment, I heard extensive moralizing about the Joffes and how they pushed the boundaries of "appropriate" parenting. The anthropologist Mary Ellen MacDonald and the nursing scholar Mary Ann Murray have persuasively argued that in clinical discourse, the word "appropriate" functions as a moral technology. Rather than expressing dispassionate clinical judgment, they suggest, the term can be used to legitimize "personal opinion under the guise of unbiased scientific certainty."[24] At times, a clinical judgment of appropriateness also reflected a class bias. For example, Dr. Petrosian characterized as inappropriate the fact that an eleven-year-old patient slept in the same room as her mother because she frequently became dizzy and her mother helped her to the bathroom in the middle of the night. However, it was not clear that there was another place for the mother to sleep, because there were already six people (two grandparents and two younger siblings, in addition to patient and mother) living in a three-bedroom house. Judgments regarding appropriateness might thus reflect a lack of sensitivity to the local contexts of families' lives.

This is not to say, however, that judgments about family dynamics were always at odds with families' own sensibilities. Anne Rothschild, the mother of West Clinic patient Brandon Rothschild, credited a pediatric neurologist for prompting her to dig into her husband's extramarital affair following a rather bluntly framed clinical inquiry about where Brandon's father was. In the end, Anne conceded that their marital discord likely had played a role in Brandon's headaches, and was grateful for the prompt. This example serves as a helpful reminder that clinicians' moral judgments, harsh they may seem, may nevertheless accord with families' own versions of reality.

## CULTURAL DILEMMAS OF DEPENDENCY AND CARE

Deliberations about appropriate parental behavior also raise cultural dilemmas of dependency. The idea of codependency—manipulation by someone else's needs—has a long history in U.S. popular and clinical psychology,[25] and its specter looms especially large in pediatric pain medicine. Clinicians on the pain team often spoke of *enmeshment,* a psychological term used to denote an unhealthy form of familial interdependency, suggesting that it is possible to care *too* well. As Rebecca Hunter put it, when I asked about the West Clinic families, "They tend to be, um, invested in their kids. I mean, sometimes overly, which is why a lot of them have pain. But at least they care. Their intentions are almost always good."

Sometimes, this discourse surpassed the merely unhealthy and veered into the explicitly pathological, as when clinicians toyed with the diagnostic label of Münchausen's syndrome by proxy, a psychological disorder in which a caregiver fabricates or exaggerates the symptoms of a loved one because she benefits from the attention received from medical providers. Although such serious allegations were rarely leveled directly, clinicians often spoke of what Rebecca Lester has called an "attenuated form of Münchausen's."[26] As one physician from outside the West Clinic put it, "Sometimes it goes to such an extent that I refer to it as a Münchausen's-by-proxy kind of phenomenon. . . . She's not cutting the child or poisoning them or something like that, which is the overt Münchausen's by proxy from a medical point of view. But it's Münchausen's by proxy in that the mother has a need for the child to have pain and psychologically perpetuates a dependent state to feed her own psychopathology."[27]

The frequent use of the Münchausen's label in the West Clinic's backstage clinical discourse points to the multiple forms of familial abuse and pathology that circulated in the pain team's diagnostic imaginary. Some parents were likewise aware of the possibility that their behavior could be read in this way. One mother I interviewed, a former nurse, expressed a fear that, due to frequent emergency room trips for her daughter's mysterious symptoms, hospital staff would perceive her as a candidate for a diagnosis of Münchausen's by proxy.

However, clinical frames for intimacy and interdependence can gloss over the multiple, ambivalent meanings of family care, pathologizing seemingly aberrant kinship ties as perverse attachments.[28] Moreover, despite significant concerns about parental overinvolvement, *inattentiveness* to children's needs is the flipside of the coin of adolescent dependency. When I asked Laurel Handelman about the dynamics among West Clinic families, she responded that while the parents of younger children had a tendency to be overprotective, with the older adolescents, "You see more of the kid who's adultified. And feels more responsible for the parents." Laurel saw a clear connection between such dynamics and the development of chronic pain: "If you think about it, the pain kind of would bring this young person to the role of being taken care of."

This dual-edged sword of adolescent dependency raises the issue of double bind, a long-standing trope in cultural anthropology. The anthropologist Gregory Bateson has defined a double bind as an emotionally distressing situation in which an individual receives multiple conflicting messages from a valued other, such that she cannot possibly respond to one set of injunctions without negating another one. The end result is that actors must choose between incompatible alternatives, necessarily resulting in disappointment.[29] Because Bateson initially posed double-bind theory as a communicative account of schizophrenia, he was particularly attuned to the ways in which clinical expectations pose contradictory demands that may interfere with recovery.

West Clinic parents were caught in a powerful double bind, insofar as they were expected to do a lot for their children—schedule appointments, transport them back and forth, pay for uncovered services, and attend therapy sessions themselves—while still keeping their distance and encouraging their children's autonomy.[30] This left them in the precarious position of being both targets of intervention and therapeutic agents. However critical the team might have been of overinvolved parents—and I heard countless offhand comments about patients who needed "bilateral parentectomies,"[31] I heard just as many criticisms of parents whom the team viewed as aloof or indifferent. In fact, both of these critiques were leveled at the Joffes: early in Claire's treatment, the team charged that Ricky was intrusive and overprotective, but later on he and Trish were criticized for leaving Claire to call her pediatrician or being late to pick her up. Consequently, it is difficult to see how the Joffes might have responded "appropriately" to clinical expectations of parental behavior.

These contradictory critiques of mundane family practices illustrate that dependency is at stake for American families in ways that transcend the purely clinical. Such conflictive readings of parental behavior follow families in and out of various types of institutional settings—for example, in schools, or even in the courts. Therefore, contrary to certain sociological interpretations that easily fit parenting styles into race and class categories,[32] my own work suggests that professional interpretations of parents' intentions can be contested, evolving, and uncertain. This is particularly likely when the cultural values that animate family practices and professional (mis)readings are already ambivalent and fraught. The ambiguous status of dependency in American culture reverberates throughout this clinical ethnography, illustrating deeply embedded anxieties about social relations of care.

This chapter has thus illustrated that explanatory frameworks for pediatric pain reveal deeply held assumptions about normative family life. Yet adolescents are embedded in broader societal structures just as assuredly as they are embedded in families. In the next chapter, I turn to explanations of pediatric pain that attribute blame at the societal level.

# Locating Pain in Societal Stress

Without civilization there can be no nervousness; there is no
race, no climate, no environment that can make nervousness
and nervous disease possible and common save when
re-enforced by brain-work and worry and in-door life.

—George M. Beard, *American Nervousness: Its Causes and
Consequences*

Careers are important. What's gonna get you a lot of money.

—Michael Harris, West Clinic patient

The first thing that I learned about eleven-year-old Brittany Rogers was
a telling admission that she had printed in thin, wavering letters on the
pain clinic's intake questionnaire: "Middle school stresses me out."
Brittany, a petite ballet dancer and straight-A student with straw-
colored hair and very pale skin, had been suffering from stomachaches
and migraines for six months at the time of her first visit to the pain
clinic. Brittany indicated that her heavy course load in California's
GATE (Gifted and Talented Education) program at her public middle
school was a primary source of stress. She spent four to six hours nightly
on her homework, and often worried that she wouldn't be able to finish
it. She also knew that she would have to go to summer school if she got
two "unsatisfactory" marks on her report card—a major cause for concern, even though it did not seem (to me) that this was likely. Brittany
was in advanced math—pre-algebra—and if she maintained her A, she
would enroll in eighth-grade math as a seventh grader.

At her first appointment, Dr. Novak told Brittany that her neurobiology—that of a bright, motivated, and capable, if somewhat over-
whelmed, adolescent—had put her at risk for developing chronic pain

problems, but it would also enable her to learn strategies to cope with the pain. Therefore, in addition to prescribing two medications, Celexa and Neurontin, Dr. Novak recommended Iyengar yoga with Tess Bergman and hypnotherapy with Charlotte LeFevre. The hypnotherapy, Dr. Novak explained, would help Brittany to learn strategies to "change the circuitry in her brain."

Initially, Brittany and her mother, Jane, were concerned about how Brittany's father would react to the part of Dr. Novak's explanatory model that linked Brittany's pain to her smartness, and, implicitly, her academic stress. Both Brittany and Jane viewed Brittany's father as a major source of pressure. Jane noted that her husband had not attended college (though she herself had) and that as a result, he had high aspirations for his daughter. Although Jane acknowledged that some of Brittany's perfectionism was self-driven, she also added, "My husband likes her to get straight A's. It's part of our family dynamic, for sure." At first, then, Brittany and Jane opted not to tell him about Dr. Novak's explanation because they worried that he might view it as a personal indictment. "He really hates to be wrong," Brittany explained. "So we didn't really tell him 'cause we were kind of a little bit afraid that he would be really angry."

From the outset, Jane's husband had been skeptical about bringing Brittany to the West Clinic because its therapeutic orientation emphasized pain management rather than cure. The news that there would be no more tests, that they were essentially "stuck" with the pain, had been hard for him to accept. However, Jane recalled, "Once we got some skills, like the yoga and stuff, then he felt like, oh, he could say, well, she would do a pose, she would try [something]. It gave him a little bit more, um, a few more ways to deal with it." Brittany became a model patient, practicing her therapeutic skills diligently. "When I got a headache," she observed, "I would just do the pose and the headache would completely go away." She also responded positively to the clinicians' suggestion that stress played a role in her pain, and gradually relinquished her perfectionism. She explained, "Before I would have to make sure that everything is perfect, like it has to be the best in the world. But now I just kind of figure that it's not the most important thing. That we don't have to spend that much time on it."

Thus far, we have seen how pediatric pain clinicians employ neurobiological explanatory frames to explain puzzling symptoms and legitimize patients' suffering. We have also seen, in turn, how the interpretive work of chronic illness outstrips these neurobiological frames, revealing more complex and shifting targets of personal responsibility and family blame. In this chapter, I turn my attention to the final tier in this explanatory trilogy, which is hinted at in Brittany Rogers's story: societal explanations for pain.

As with earlier chapters, the prototypical West Clinic patient as smart, successful, and overburdened is a central trope in the pages that follow. Here, however, the focus is shifted slightly to explore the ways in which ideas about the culture of stress in the contemporary United States generate explanatory frames that favor societal causality. In examining such claims about the sociogenic nature of illness, I situate the experience of West Clinic patients within a broader conversation about American adolescence, which the early twentieth-century developmental psychologist G. Stanley Hall famously characterized, in the first textbook devoted to the topic, as a period of "storm and stress."[1] For some adolescents, I argue here, chronic patienthood offered a pathway out of a stressful life and a welcome opportunity to reimagine aspirational futures.

The idea that chronic pain might in some way be caused by societal stress has its roots in a long line of cultural and historical narratives that have linked illness to rapid social change and the pressures of modernity In her 2008 book *The Cure Within: A History of Mind-Body Medicine*, the historian Anne Harrington examines the emergence in the late-nineteenth-century United States of a theory of psychosomatic illness that framed those afflicted as "broken by modern life." Harrington traces this narrative back to the New York neurologist George M. Beard, who used the term *neurasthenia* to describe a cluster of symptoms (fatigue, anxiety, headache, and depression) hypothesized to result from the depletion of the central nervous system's energy reserves.[2] Beard attributed neurasthenia, which seemed to affect the wealthy and educated disproportionately, to the strains wrought by modern civilization, particularly urbanization and associated changes in occupational life. The condition was primarily experienced "in civilized, intellectual communities" and served as "part of the compensation for our progress and our refinement."[3] Beard dubbed it a uniquely American disease and attributed it to the harsh American climate and the fast pace of American life. Treatment, which typically included an extended vacation of sorts in the American wilderness (for men) or a lengthy dose of bed rest (for women), permitted the afflicted temporarily to escape the stresses of modern life.

By the mid twentieth century, the diagnosis of neurasthenia had fallen out of favor in the United States,[4] but it was soon replaced with another enduring cultural index: the Type A personality.[5] Whereas the central feature of neurasthenia was exhaustion, the rise of the Type A personality marked an emerging concern with *stress*. The concept of stress, as an explanation for bodily symptoms, was first popularized in the aftermath of World War I and the experience of shell shock. The shift from nerves to stress was significant because the concept of "nerves" located illness within an individual body, while the concept of stress offered, at least on the surface, a new way to externalize physical symptoms to forms of social pathology.[6] However, the practical meanings of stress have mutated over the years, and it has come to signify, in some cases, a superficial and incomplete means of folding decontextualized "social" characteristics into behavioral analysis.[7]

A defining feature of the popular discourse on stress in the contemporary United States is a tension between individual and societal levels of explanation. Stress is at once the product of the fast pace of modern life and the failure of individuals to adapt to this environment. Consequently, there is an overriding ambivalence about where to locate responsibility for adolescent stress: with society for imposing unrealistic expectations on contemporary adolescents, or with the adolescents themselves who internalize and even amplify these demands. Despite this chapter's emphasis on explanations of pain leveraged at the level of society, then, the typical patient as a specific figure "at risk" for chronic pain remains very much in the foreground in the pages that follow. Clinicians outspokenly criticized the level of stress facing adolescents in contemporary American society, even as the antidotes positioned pain at the level of individual responsibility and blame. As I will show, the specific configuration of the relationship between the person and society is very much at stake in explanations of chronic pain.

## AMERICAN ADOLESCENCE AND THE CULTURE OF STRESS

In his penetrating book *Producing Success: The Culture of Personal Advancement in an American High School,* the anthropologist Peter Demerath notes that it might easily have become an "ethnography of stress," since "that is where the voices, experiences, and concerns of so many of these upwardly oriented young people . . . led us."[8] The students that Demerath observed lived hyperscheduled lives, were tired all of the time, and evinced what he viewed as an unhealthy obsession with success. This description resonates unmistakably with my own observations in the West Clinic. Many, if not most, of the patients were enrolled in GATE programs and a large number of them in honors and AP classes. Most were involved in several sports and in clubs, music, dance, and other creative activities as well. They engaged in such pursuits both for recreational purposes and for their instrumental value in college admissions. The pressure to succeed was a pervasive force in their social networks, and the propensity to measure one's success by attending a competitive college was ubiquitous.

While scholars and cultural critics alike have observed that high-school students in many privileged and affluent areas of the United States live under an enormous amount of everyday stress,[9] what is particularly striking about the historical moment in which my research was set is that traditional middle-class goals like attending a good college ceased to offer a surefire way of ensuring future success. As newspaper headlines during this time touted alarming numbers of unemployed humanities majors, college became an unstable object of middle-class aspiration: with popular attention turning increasingly to the value of education in STEM fields, merely going to college was no longer enough. This is not to say that adolescents living in other cultural and socioeconomic contexts do not face obvious daily challenges,[10] but rather that the popular discourse on stress in the contemporary United States is inflected with certain class-based assumptions about work, civic engagement, and future aspirations.

Michael Harris, whose case is discussed in chapter 2, reflected these sentiments as he mused to me about his future plans. He had been thinking about the military, he said, but was now shifting his attention toward science: "Careers are important. What's gonna get you a lot of money. . . . so you can support a family if you have one. What can get you a car and gas, what can feed yourself. So you've gotta think about those before you go with what you wanna [do]." Michael's remarks reveal a precocious awareness that when thinking about a career path, it is important to consider what jobs will offer security for oneself and one's family.

Such concerns were all too real for Michael, whose father, a firefighter, was about to go back to school to become an emergency medical technician at the time that these remarks were made. Rob's career shift was motivated primarily by the prospect of earning more. Although he had made the decision to go back to school before Michael's pain developed, the cost of Michael's treatment had taken a substantial toll on the family.

Rob told me, early in Michael's treatment, that Dr. Sterling charged $300 an hour, and the first appointment was set for a two-hour timeslot; he was hoping to recover 40 percent of this from his insurance company, but was not certain that he would. "What choice do we have?" Rob reflected. He reasoned that they were lucky to be able to do it, and if he picked up an extra day of work, he could pay for a month of Michael's treatments. On the other hand, he acknowledged, he had not been able to do any overtime work since Michael's ordeal had begun, because he needed to be more available for supervision and appointments.

In light of the grim economic climate, many of the patients I interviewed reported concerns about burdening their families with the cost of their treatment. Such anxieties were clearly borne out in their parents' testimonies—and by the occasional bounced check that I heard of in team meetings. For many adolescents in the West Clinic, these anxieties played a fundamental role in a broader culture of stress that shaped their pain experience in critical, if sometimes oblique, ways. To be clear, I am not suggesting that clinicians, parents, or patients themselves believed that the pain was *directly* produced by social and economic uncertainty. Rather, I am arguing that such pain is polyvalent, expressing broader rifts in the social order along with more individualized— and individualizing—causes. In doing so, I consider how stress gives specific shape to the social contours of the painful body, amplifying certain meanings of embodied distress.[11]

Another way of approaching the problem of how to configure the relationship between pain and stress is to ask: if pain medicine is the tool, what is the object of intervention? What, in other words, are we medicating? The significance of these questions was made clear to me by an exchange that I observed on an August day in the West Clinic. The mother of a fourteen-year-old patient, Ryan, told Dr. Petrosian that they had come "to throw ourselves at your mercy": to write more prescriptions for the powerful painkillers that Ryan was on—OxyContin, oxycodone, and several others—to get him through the beginning of the school year. Thanks to this medication, Ryan's mother noted, they had just come back from their first "worry-free" vacation since the preceding October, and, she said, "We have hope for the first time in so long." Ryan himself appeared incredibly nervous throughout the interaction, rubbing his hands through his hair and wiping his face repeatedly. Somewhat reluctantly, Dr. Petrosian agreed to write the prescriptions, but he only provided a month's worth of pills, without any refills, so that they could reevaluate how Ryan was doing at the end of that period.

Back in the chart room, Dr. Petrosian told me that he thought that we would be seeing more and more kids like Ryan. When I asked him what he meant, he cited Ryan's tremendous anxiety. "Kids today are under such enormous pressure, and this is the result," he said pensively. From this perspective, chronic pain is as much a logical response to a "sick society" as a neurobiological problem, and pain medication intervenes in the culture of adolescent stress as much as in individual bodies. This social diagnosis was not intended to suggest that Ryan's pain was not real. Rather, it highlights how multiple forms of distress shape the cultural meaning of pain.

### Stress and Illness Causality

Whereas neurobiological explanations for pain were most likely to appear in initial conversations with families, and team meetings were especially conducive to psychoanalytic explanations, societal explanations for pain were most prevalent in my interviews with clinicians. In understanding why this was so, it may be useful to think of the anthropological interview as yet another "stage" on which clinicians performed. Outside of the intimate setting of the clinic, the interview formed a particularly suitable stage for expressing explanatory narratives that made sense of embodied distress via interpretive frames that transcended the individual and the clinical. In other words, this stage offered a fitting arena for clinicians to voice larger social grievances, and in doing so, to point to the limits of clinical interventions to resolve pediatric pain.

In interviews, clinicians expressed multiple theories regarding the sources of adolescent stress. Some blamed the recent onslaught of state-mandated educational testing and a growing culture of competition for fostering unnecessary pressure. Dr. Petrosian explained, "You know, it's an 'everyone's gotta be a winner' society. And I don't want to be that second-place guy by myself with all these first-place kids in front of me. Like it's a minority all of a sudden to be in second place. There is no third place—it's like, 'Oh my gosh, I'm in second place. It's lonely up on this second pedestal for the silver medal with these forty guys on the gold medal plate,' you know."

There was also widespread agreement that parents played an important role. "I think that a lot of these families put a lot of pressure on these kids for success. And doing well in school," Rebecca Hunter told me one afternoon in the tranquil setting of her home office. She acknowledged that the pressure did not always come from the parents: "I have plenty of parents that say, 'I don't know where this comes from.' That's like how I was growing up. It did not come from my parents at all. They were like hippies. I mean, they're very educated and very smart, but they didn't put any pressure on me at all, and I was totally self-driven. And so I get that, when parents say, 'I swear it's not coming from me.' I even—I believe them. . . . but a lot of times it is."

Rebecca's explanation made sense to me because it captured my own experience to a certain extent. I was fortunate enough to attend a highly ranked public school in an affluent suburban city, where I worked extremely hard—much harder, in fact, than I did until I got to graduate school. At the time, I denied that my parents had pressured me to take a heavy load of honors courses and get accepted into an elite college. It was only many years later that I came to appreciate the tacit ways in which my family had shaped the academic culture that I grew up in, regardless of whether I experienced a tangible sense of pressure.

I recall an anthropologist colleague looking at me with raised eyebrows, for example, when right after describing my father's annual practice of calculating the percentage of seniors in my high school's graduating class who would be attending an Ivy League college in the fall, I claimed that my motivation to succeed was entirely self-driven. (That my high-school newspaper printed the future plans of each graduating class, enabling such a calculus, is another matter entirely.) The social theorist Pierre Bourdieu might say that the pressure on high-achieving adolescents like the West Clinic patients and myself is so internalized that it masks the relations of power that shape the embodied dispositions of those who occupy a particular social status, or what Bourdieu has called *habitus*.

If the various sources of pressure were somewhat obscured, however, it was eminently clear that this pressure began at a very young age. The physical therapist Meg Pratt, who blamed the schools more than other clinicians I spoke with, spoke of a patient who had already internalized the pressure to attend a good college, although she was only eight: "I was explaining to her about stress. And how different things can cause stress. Basically anything that causes you to adapt or change can be stressful. . . . And I said, 'Sometimes it's stressful when you're trying to—when you want to get an A and you feel stressed when you get a B on a test.' And I said, 'But it's really not life-threatening if you get a B on a test.' And she said, 'Oh yes it is.' This is a kid in elementary school," Meg said, with an air of disbelief.

Meg continued, animating her young patient's account: "'If you don't get an A on all your tests, than you're not going to get an A at the end of the semester. And if you don't get all A's at your school, then you're not going to get into the better private school. And if you don't get into the better private school and get good grades, then you're not going to get into the top universities in the United States. And if you don't get into the top university in the United States, then you're not gonna be as successful in life.' She was eight! Eight years old . . . what a horrible thing for a child to have that amount of stress." In this account, stress is configured as an internal pressure to succeed, which is further linked to the desire to attend a top university, a specific marker of academic success that is highly salient in middle-class American communities. From this perspective, stress is not a demand for physical labor, but a sustained anxiety surrounding mental work.

Busy schedules and academic demands were not the only sources of stress facing West Clinic patients, however. Some reported troubles ranging from social isolation to teasing to overt bullying. Michael Harris and his parents viewed his long-term bullying by middle-school peers as a direct cause of his stomachaches. As Michael so eloquently put it, "In [my school] the social ladder is missing a few links." When I asked him to elaborate, he replied, "It's almost like in those movies where they're crossing the old bridge. One wrong step and the entire bridge collapses. . . . The only time you're safe is when you're at the tippy tip-top. And then you get to control what everyone else does. So you stomp on the top and everyone starts shaking." If attending school each day was for Michael an exercise in navigating a rickety social structure, stomachaches and depression were the fallout of this unstable existence.

How, exactly, did this happen? Rebecca Hunter offered what I would call a hydraulic model, in which stress is conceptualized as a physical pressure that accumulates within the body. The longer it remains "bottled up," the more the pressure swells, until it must eventually find a way out. West Clinic patients thus externalize their stress through pain symptoms. Rebecca described how she might explain this process to a patient:

I explain to most of my kids that if their body is like a jar, and they're stuffing their emotions into it—'cause I think a lot of pain comes from not expressing sadness and anger, or what we call negative emotions. If they're stuffing them into the jar, and the lid is on the jar, and they keep stuffing them in, eventually it's gonna explode. You know, it's gonna explode through a pain disorder, through blowing up [in] anger, or it's gonna—or some of our kids who just crash and can't get up for months. I mean literally. . . . But I said, if you poke even just a couple little holes in it every day, just a little bit, just enough to let it ooze out a little bit, it will never actually explode.

In other words, as several clinicians observed, whereas some adolescents "act out" and rebel, the prototypical West Clinic patient "acts in." Rebecca elaborated on this distinction: "I think the kids who are rebelling and who are not really so in tune with everybody else's needs and not worried about taking care of their parents and stuff, they don't have that—they don't internalize that pressure. So I think if it comes out, it's not gonna stay in the body. It stays in the body with these kids [West Clinic patients] because they're holding all this stuff in." This line of thought thus suggests that West Clinic patients express distress through the body because other expressive channels elude them.[12]

In Rebecca's hydraulic model, "holding in" the stress was conceptualized as a relatively passive process, even though many patients who dropped out of school and other activities as a result of their pain came to welcome these changes. Occasionally, however, clinicians suggested that patients were "holding on" to pain in more intentional ways. At one team meeting, the clinicians praised an eighteen-year-old patient who was, in their view, holding on to her pain as a way to avoid a college athletics scholarship, which they believed her parents had forced her into. In cases such as this one, chronic pain appeared to enable adolescents to rationalize decisions that would be otherwise difficult to make, raising questions about agency and resistance, themes that I return to at the end of the chapter.

If dropping out of certain activities offered a temporary respite from the stresses and strains of adolescent life, reintegration after a prolonged absence could also pose challenges, and it often provoked a relapse. "School has very often been a trigger," Charlotte LeFevre told me. "As you've heard in the group, 'Oh, she was fine until she went back to school.'" This was certainly the case for Claire Joffe, whose symptoms briefly resurfaced when she returned to school for her tenth-grade year. Some West Clinic patients were never able to make a full return to school.

In what follows, I offer three portraits of West Clinic patients that highlight different dimensions of the relationship between stress, social pressures, and pain. The first such case involves an exceptionally bright and ambitious seventeen-year-old girl who was not able to return to high school after an accident that left her with chronic headaches.

Chronic pain drove her off the track to an elite university, giving her a way out of a highly stressful lifestyle and an opportunity to fashion a very different sort of life for herself.

## LILA FELDMAN

In October of her junior year of high school, Lila Feldman flew to Atlanta with her parents to attend a cousin's bat mitzvah. She hadn't wanted to go. "I was bogged down," she said. "I was basically running around with my head cut off." At the time, Lila was taking five AP courses, playing the violin in three different orchestras, and being trained to compete in her school's academic decathlon. To make the trip, she would need to miss a day of school, and with a test coming up soon, she was anxious about missing calculus. "Even though it's this big family thing that's really important, I was like, 'I cannot miss school,' you know?" she told me, laughing as she relayed the story. Fifteen months later, her circumstances had changed enough for her to recognize her shortsightedness.

On the morning of the bat mitzvah, Lila slipped and fell out of the hotel shower, landing on the toilet. She recalled: "I remember as I was falling, I was twisting around, and I looked towards the wall and there was nothing to grab onto." Although she bruised the entire side of her face, she did not think much of the fall initially. "You know, I'm a klutz. I fall *all* the time," she told me. She went to the ceremony and the party that night, and got on the plane to return home the next day. "*That's* when it started hurting," Lila explained. "It felt like someone was trying to um, claw their way out of my head. Like, who was it, was born out of Zeus's head? It was Athena, I think?"

When Lila awoke the next morning, she couldn't get out of bed. Yet she couldn't sleep, either. Everything hurt. Her mother sent her to school, but she came back home right away, because "the bell had rung and I had like, *freaked* out" at the piercing sound. The next day, Lila's pediatrician ordered a CT scan, to make sure that she had not sustained damage from the fall, but everything appeared fine. The doctor also prescribed medication, but it did little to help her all-over body pain, migraines, and dizziness, not to mention her overwhelming exhaustion and sensitivity to light and sound.

Despite feeling lousy, Lila tried to return to school. Junior year was an important year for college preparation, and she had started to look for teachers to write her letters of recommendation. When I asked Mimi, Lila's mother, what was going on in Lila's life at the time of the accident, she said, "Oh my god. Right before, we were looking at colleges." Lila noted, "I've been groomed for college my entire life." Lila's father, a teacher, was particularly keen for her to make a swift return to her regular routine. Mimi maintained that they were not "pushy parents," an assessment that Lila concurred with, but Mimi discovered after Lila's injury that her husband Joseph "was *way* more attached to the whole achievement issue." She found this surprising, given Joseph's "anti-establishment" leanings. "You know, he's like a child of the sixties and I'm like, right at the tail [end of that decade] as well. So it kind of shocked me." As a result, Mimi said, "He had more, I think, to let go of than I did."

When Lila fell down the stairs at school following a wave of dizziness, even Joseph conceded that a break might be in order. Yet when they started to investigate home-study options, Lila realized that she could not read for more than five minutes at a time without her headaches getting worse. Barely sleeping and barely eating, Lila grew frail and pale. "My parents called me Vampyra," she recalled. "'Cause I'd stay up all night, like a bat in the belfry." Things continued this way for the rest of the academic year, which was especially hard for Joseph. Lila explained, "We got in a lot of arguments 'cause he'd try to force me to go to school. And I'd tell him that I didn't feel well enough, and he'd of course, you know, say, like, 'Well if you want to stay here 'til you're thirty-five, that's your business.'" Meanwhile, Joseph's own parents were struggling with addictions to spending and getting into trouble with debt. Mimi spoke of this period wistfully: "Our family just became so *sad*. It just, uh, you know, everything became . . . you know we were living in this, like, cloud of sadness, I guess."

Lila began seeing a neurologist, who diagnosed her with postconcussion syndrome, and a rheumatologist, who diagnosed her with secondary fibromyalgia, but her progress was slow, and she remained in bed for much of the time. Finally, in August, Mimi's own therapist asked her to speak with a palliative care physician, who told her about the West Clinic. At Dr. Petrosian's recommendation, Lila began doing hypnotherapy with Charlotte, which helped her sleep, and yoga with Tess, which helped her regain her strength.

Lila's treatment took a toll on the family both financially and emotionally. Mimi explained, "It was hard because, you know, traffic's really bad, and, you know, and I have a home office, you know, I'm supposed to be working. And everything's out of pocket, nothing is covered by insurance." Responsibility for shuttling Lila back and forth from therapy sessions fell largely to Mimi because, as a lawyer employed by the state, she had a more flexible work schedule than that of her husband, a teacher. Finances were already a concern because Mimi's pay was contingent upon the state budget, and the prior summer she hadn't been paid for four months when the budget did not pass. With Lila's injury, Mimi had to scale back her work even further because she spent so much time driving Lila around to therapy sessions. She noted that this was "not good financially," but that "we had savings, which was good." She also felt fortunate to have a flexible job: "I mean, if you had a regular job, you'd have to quit or something. I don't know how you would actually do it, really, you know?"

In the team meetings, the clinicians described Lila as "smart," "over-extended," and "Stanford-bound," the kind of kid that was "push push push." But it was Charlotte's description of Lila as "one of our kids" that initially captured my attention. When I interviewed Charlotte, she elaborated on what this meant: "Generally we'll say, 'Oh, they're one of our kids.' Meaning that they're high-achieving kids, push really hard, maybe push too hard. And their body just finally says, 'Mm mm. No more. You're gonna slow down.'" This description highlights the ambivalence that the West Clinic staff exhibited toward the role of stress in pain causality. Although they often charged parents, schools, and society at large with putting unhealthy pressure on adolescents to succeed, they also conceptualized stress at the level of the individual body, suggesting that some adolescents did not take proper care of themselves. In many cases, then, it was hard to determine whether adolescents were "pushing too hard," as in Charlotte's framing, or rather being "pushed" by external forces that they had little power to control.

Aware that her treatment was costing her parents a lot of money, Lila was motivated by a feeling that "Well, I better make this worth it, you know?" While she committed herself to yoga and hypnotherapy, she was less enthusiastic about her medication. She told me that she hated taking Celexa, which Dr. Petrosian had prescribed to help her sleep. She explained, "I just really don't like the idea that my feelings aren't my own." Describing herself as a "purist," Lila noted that when sick, she typically drank herbal tea and went to sleep.

Slowly, things improved for Lila. However, when the team tried to help her transition back to school at the beginning of the new academic year, she relapsed. She told me later that fall, "It turns out being in school is actually harder than schoolwork. Just being around people. Like there were times when I'd go to school and I'd be like, in front of the classroom about to go into class when this *obnoxious* girl would come and like scream to her friends down below the stairs." Such disruptions would send Lila, still extremely sensitive to auditory stimulation, to the nurse's office, undone for the day.

This extreme sensitivity provoked a backstage concern about whether Lila might be "sticky." At a team meeting early in Lila's treatment, Tess Bergman remarked that every once in a while, Lila seemed to display signs of being on the PDD spectrum. She relayed how Lila had recently started walking through the hallways at school with her backpack worn in front and her boyfriend shielding her so that no one would bump into her. Lila herself sometimes referred to her "odd wiring," an idiom that she used to make sense of her social peculiarities and distinctive worldview.

Gradually, Lila and her parents lowered their expectations for a return to school. "At first I was like, 'Gotta get back! Gotta get back!'" she remembered. "And, um, now I'm kinda like, 'Phew.' Now, you know. Glad that's over." Lila told Rebecca Hunter that it had been as if she were running on a hamster's wheel, spinning, and couldn't get off. She needed to crash in order to stop. Lila was not able to return to her violin playing, either. She said, "I haven't played in over a year now. It's kind of sad, but at the same time, that is a really low priority."

Perhaps more significantly, Lila also let go of her long-term dream of going to Stanford. Unable to enroll in a home-schooling program due to her continued difficulties with reading, she realized that she would have to make up two years of high school in order to get her diploma. She resigned herself to attending community college the following fall, after which she could transfer into the University of California system (a certain number of slots were guaranteed to students from local community colleges). Without a high-school diploma, Lila could not apply to Stanford.

It saddened Mimi that her daughter had so easily given up such a long-standing dream. She reflected, "Of course when she has been dealing with a lot of pain it's really easy for us to let go of, you know, the academic stuff that she was hoping for. I mean that is nothing to me, because, you know, I'm just wanting her to feel well. . . . But when I think about her, I still feel terrible. You know, for her. And it's such a young age, to have to deal with such loss, really, you know?" When I spoke with Lila, however, she sounded more sanguine. She told me, "So the new plan is junior college in the fall, once I turn eighteen. . . . what's really great is it's kind of like a new start. I don't have to deal with all the stresses of going back into AP, you know? Of being who I was? I'm kind of like a totally different person now."

It is difficult to parse the extent to which Lila truly embraced this opportunity to become "a totally different person," or whether she framed her story in this way to persuade herself of the merits of these alternative aspirations. As narrative theorists have argued, the temporal dimensions of personal narratives offer a powerful rhetorical tool for reshaping self-understandings and directing possible futures.[13] I knew from the team meetings that Charlotte had been actively working with Lila to help her let go of Stanford and "establish a new dream," and I saw subtle traces of this effort in the way that Lila spoke about Stanford: "I had like built in my mind that Stanford was like my dream. Well, it was. . . . But somehow in my mind I'd stacked up Stanford with happiness, like if I can get into Stanford, I can get into a good graduate school, get a career, support a family—and have a 'happy ever after' kind of thing." It is not easy to determine if Lila was trying this narrative on for size or if she had fully assimilated it.

Mimi likewise saw Lila's illness experience through the lens of a transformative journey. She suggested that Lila's circumstances had occasioned a sort of ethical conversion, an opportunity for Lila to "fashion herself in the way that she wants." Mimi explained to me, "She put herself on this really fast track. And I think she might have thought she wanted to be a doctor or something. And I'm understanding now that she doesn't really want to be a doctor, you know? So maybe whatever she does will be more—will come from more of what she wants instead of what she feels like she *should* do."

Mimi's description of Lila's illness as a critical turning point in her self-discovery resonates with a growing body of anthropological scholarship that views the therapeutic process as an opportunity for transforming one's moral personhood.[14] Yet if such transformation was an essential component of the therapeutic process, it was so because there was something about Lila's old way of life that was no longer sustainable. Lila's headaches exempted her from school, her orchestras, and the like, effectively suspending her stressful existence, and she took refuge in the sick role. In fact, following her illness, her daily pursuits mirrored those recommended by physicians for early twentieth-century neurasthenics: she spent her days working on needlepoint and doing what she called "granny things."

The sociologist Talcott Parsons introduced the concept of the sick role to elucidate the reciprocal obligations between a sick person and society. Drawing on a functionalist framework, Parsons stipulated that sickness is a form of "sanctioned deviance," and that, as a social role, it comes with certain expectations and responsibilities.[15] But if for Parsons the goal of the sick role was to return sick people to normal functioning, Lila Feldman's case illustrates that chronically ill people do not generally return to their preexisting social roles. Instead, they find ways to accommodate prior obligations to new circumstances, renegotiating social relationships and responsibilities along the way. From this perspective, the sick role does not serve to maintain a preexisting social order, but rather gives way to a new sense of normalcy.

It appeared that Lila had in a sense been "broken by modern life," and that assembling a new aspirational future was a major achievement of her therapy in the West Clinic. From my perspective, Lila did seem happier with the slower pace of life she found after her injury. She seemed to genuinely appreciate time spent at home, alone, or with her dog and her boyfriend. However, because I had not observed Lila's therapeutic interactions with Charlotte, it remained somewhat unclear to me how much work had gone into selling Lila on this new way of life.

## ELI LERNER

When I asked Eli Lerner about the cause of his pain, he responded simply: "Stress. More stress, more leg pain." On the face of it, this response sounded similar to that of other high-achieving clinic patients, like Lila Feldman and Brittany Rogers. However, underlying this seemingly straightforward narrative was a more complex account of family troubles and socioeconomic hardship. Perhaps more than other families in my study, the Lerner family epitomized the precarious economic situation of the American middle class during the late oos. Eli's father, Ravi, had run a small computer repair company for twenty-two years when one of his clients offered him a permanent job. Ravi accepted, but he had recently been laid off from the job when I met the family. Since then, Ravi had been trying to grow his business again, an unpromising proposition in light of the ongoing recession at the time. Eli's mother, Elsa, had done the accounting for the family business, but she had recently taken a temporary job doing medical filing.

The first time that I met Eli in the West Clinic, he told me that he wanted to become a screenwriter. Eli had developed chronic pain more than three years earlier, during his freshman year of high school, and his high-school career had been punctuated by prolonged absences and intermittent homeschooling, but his commitment to writing never faltered. Prior to his freshman year, Eli had attended a private Jewish school, and the switch to public school had been difficult. Most of his friends were attending a Jewish high school in the area, but the tuition was expensive—$19,000 the first year and $20,000 each subsequent year—and his parents had not received enough financial aid for Eli to attend. Eli found the classes at his high school "stale" and unchallenging, and some of his classmates teased him because he wore a *kippah* (yarmulke). "I sort of became very—I don't know if snobbish [is the right word], but like, I thought I was better than other people," he said. He began to dread going to school, and even imagined getting sick so that he could miss a week of classes, which was prescient, in a sense, because he ended up missing much more than one week.

Eli's pain began on Halloween night, when he went to a local movie theater to see a science fiction film with his sister and father. As he recounted it to me:

> [T]here was an escalator and I was running up the escalator. And I don't know if my shoes were untied or if I was just klutzy, but I fell on my knee and it was bleeding a little. But it hurt a lot. And then course I had to sit through the movie 'cause we were already there. . . . I remember limping to the car—and then I was able to limp on it—but by the end of the night, I couldn't walk on it. I couldn't even limp on it. It felt like—it felt almost like whenever I stepped on it, this sounds weird, but like a bolt of lightning shooting up my leg. It was like a brief flash of pain.

The next day, Elsa took him to his pediatrician, who diagnosed a sprained ankle. When Eli was still in pain after four weeks, he went to see an orthopedist who put his foot in a boot. At his second visit, the orthopedist told Eli that he might have reflex sympathetic dystrophy (RSD).[16] By February, Eli was still unable to walk on his foot and had not returned to school. Because he had complained so much about school during the period just before his injury, his father and four sisters were skeptical about the extent of his pain. "Even my mom was doubting me," he recalled. "It wasn't just good enough that I knew it. It really upset me and people didn't believe me. And they thought I wasn't really in pain. It's upsetting. There's no, there's no bruise, there's no bone jutting out, there's no bone, so people think, looks like there's nothing wrong, [so] there must be nothing wrong."

Finally, Eli was referred to Dr. Joseph Stanley, a pediatric pain specialist who had trained under Dr. Novak and was running another pediatric pain program in the area. Eli described Dr. Stanley as a "one-of-a-kind" doctor. At his clinic, Eli said, "They gave us reasons why, they talked to us, they related to us, they gave us proper meds." They also connected him with a local homeschooling program for children with chronic illnesses and disabilities, in which Eli was assigned a tutor who came to his house to teach him, free of charge.

Eli was homeschooled for his entire ninth-grade year. He went back to school in his sophomore year, but only made it through all six periods once. Then, on his birthday, which was also the last day of Rosh Hashanah, the mark of the Jewish New Year, he got into a terrible fight with his best friend. When his friend stormed out of the house, Eli chased after him, neglecting to use the crutches that he had come to rely on. Ravi came after Eli, and as Eli turned to walk back to his father, "I feel this upsurge. I don't know if that's the word, but this pain. And I remember—the last thing I remember was falling and my arms hitting my dad's arms." Eli fell into a seizure, convulsing and spitting up in the street.

The Lerners took Eli to an emergency room, and when he regained consciousness, he was in a tremendous amount of pain. "I remember bright lights and then I remember being on the gurney. And I also remember they were talking to me. And all of a sudden I could understand them. It was like waking up at first. And then they were gonna give me a narcotic injection but I was afraid too much. And also my parents were kind of, you know, 'It's a lot of money. It's a hundred dollars.' So they gave me one injection and it didn't work at all." Nevertheless, Eli said that the shot had worked because he didn't want his parents to have to pay more money.

The next day, Dr. Stanley called Eli, having been notified of the episode by emergency room staff. "He was not happy," Eli said. "He said that the adrenaline was running my nervous system and then when the adrenaline went away, the nervous system kind of went kaput." From Dr. Stanley's perspective, Eli should have been able to better modulate his response to the fight with his friend. I asked Eli whether he agreed with this assessment. "I don't know," he admitted. "I remember feeling this upsurge of pain, I remember feeling . . . almost like when you have to throw up and you feel it coming up. But it wasn't like vomit. It was like air. And I don't know. That's what I remember."

Eli did not go back to school after this episode, and he did not return for good until his junior year. Even then, he logged sixty absences the first semester and did not go anywhere without his cane. He also took a reduced course load, making up some of the classes over the summer.

When Dr. Stanley moved to the Midwest to start a new pain clinic, he referred Eli to the West Clinic, where he started seeing Dr. Petrosian and Meg Pratt for biofeedback and physical therapy. When I met Eli at the beginning of his senior year, his pain had clearly improved. With Meg's help, he had gotten rid of his cane and committed to a regular routine of long walks in his neighborhood, which he found therapeutic. He also took a number of medications regularly, including methadone, Lyrica, Elavil, and Lexapro. At the first of Eli's appointment with Dr. Petrosian that I observed, Eli and Elsa's primary concerns centered on the methadone. Eli reported that when he got to the end of his twelve-hour dose, he started to sweat and feel the effects of withdrawal. He wanted to try to cut back so that he would be less dependent. Dr. Petrosian encouraged him to decrease his dose as he saw fit.

Although his methadone use worried him, Eli was more amenable to long-term medication use than most West Clinic patients I spoke with. When I interviewed him later that fall, he described the effects of his meds: "I feel less depressed. I feel more confident. I feel happier a lot of the times. I don't know sometimes even just the act of taking a pill makes me feel happier, more at ease. Less stressful." He also doubted whether he would ever be able to get off of methadone permanently. "I'm worried about how my leg will feel off of it," he said. "'Cause it's like an illusion, you know, that if I have no pain for a day, it's only because I'm, you know, well-medicated." Eli did not think that the medication was curing his pain; it was only masking its effects. Consequently, he believed that he would never truly get rid of it.

At his next appointment, three months later, Eli had reduced his methadone dose from 10 mg to 5 mg. At the same time, however, owing to his family's financial constraints, he had come to rely increasingly on medication. He had begun seeing a psychiatrist, but Elsa told Dr. Petrosian that they could not return to see him until they paid the bill, which they were not in a position to do. In the meantime, she asked if Dr. Petrosian could write refills for Eli's psychiatric medications. As a stop-gap measure for much needed mental health care, Dr. Petrosian advised that Eli talk to a school counselor.

In April, when Dr. Petrosian asked how life at home was, Eli said that it was "stressful," with financial concerns pervading the household. When Dr. Petrosian commented at the same appointment that Eli's recovery would be like the stock market, with little dips along the way, Eli quipped, "I hope I'm doing better than the stock market." I had learned from Eli that his father had threatened to commit suicide after he had lost his job the year before. Eli had called the police because of these threats, which Ravi viewed as a betrayal. Eli described a complicated relationship with his father, who had grown up with what Eli described as a "rough life." During the past year, Ravi's insecurity had settled over the home like a thick fog.

By the end of Eli's senior year, most of his friends were graduating, but he did not have enough credits to walk at graduation. He planned to finish his degree at a local community college and transfer to a state university, which he described as "not a very prestigious school but it has a sentimental value 'cause my mom went there and my oldest sister went there." After that, he hoped to attend film school at the University of Southern California.

In June, Eli reported to Dr. Petrosian that he had been feeling really happy at times, wanting to do it all, and then suddenly he was uninterested in everything and lacked the energy to leave his room. Dr. Petrosian suggested that Eli return to the psychiatrist, but Elsa said, "We are totally broke and unemployed. I have to fight my husband about co-pays." Dr. Petrosian suggested that they check with Nina Herrera, the clinical coordinator, to see if there was an urgent-care psychiatric clinic Eli could go to. Then, turning to Eli, he said, "But you might need to pick up the slack on this, a bit. Get involved in activities."

When I spoke with Eli on the telephone in August, he did not mention the symptoms he had previously reported, yet things still sounded grim. He had been weaned off methadone and had had a really difficult time withdrawing. Dr. Novak, whom he had begun to see instead of Dr. Petrosian, had put him on oxycodone instead, initially just as needed, but now full-time. I didn't quite understand the logic of using oxycodone instead of methadone, since I knew that methadone was typically considered the drug of first choice to avoid opioid dependence. But Eli explained that a lot of his treatment was now being handled through e-mails with Nina, because his family had lost their insurance.

For Eli, the sick role served as a way to express discontent: with his school, his father, and the contraction of opportunities that lingered on the horizon, however optimistic he remained on the surface. Because people had commented on his creative talents throughout his life, he felt considerable pressure to succeed. "I wanna be a writer and a film director," he told me. "It's hard. People—look. People all my life [have] call[ed] me a genius, some sort of genius. And there's a thing [where] you feel like you need to live up to that."

Although Eli's daily routine did not change as dramatically as Lila's had, he also believed that his pain had changed him significantly. When I asked him how the world had changed for him, he referred me to the

1993 movie *Groundhog Day*, which stars Bill Murray as a TV weatherman who finds himself stuck in a time loop, forced to repeat the same day (Groundhog Day) over and over again. Although he finds this unbearable at first, he eventually decides to make the best of his circumstances. Eli related to Murray's character in the following way: "You know how he lives through the day and he learns piano and he becomes a better person and all that. It was like when I came back into society. I had learned guitar, I had—I'm a smarter, better person, confident, more funny, wiser."

### JASON KATZ

Both Lila Feldman and Eli Lerner acknowledged the role that stress played in the development of their chronic pain. For each of them, pain offered a form of sanctioned respite from the strains of middle-class American adolescence, and particularly the challenges of high school. But if Lila and Eli represent patients "broken by modern life," Jason Katz's story complicates received narratives about the relationship between pain and the culture of stress in American adolescence.

At the age of ten, Jason developed chronic pain in his feet, which made it difficult, and later impossible, to walk. After several consultations with orthopedists, the problem was attributed to his flat arches, and he underwent reconstructive surgery. Although the surgery was successful, the pain remained. Jason was confined to a wheelchair for two years, and his parents shuffled him around to a series of local physicians, one of whom diagnosed him with RSD and referred him to the West Clinic. When I met him, Jason was sixteen years old and had been a patient in the clinic for more than five years. By this point, his pain had spread to other areas of his body—chiefly his stomach and head, but also intermittently in his bladder, knee, and back. Jason's mother, Debbie, explained this diffusion in terms of Dr. Novak's explanatory framework for "smart neurons": "We were in Italy last year. Never had a headache in his life. Got a sinus infection. We didn't catch it soon enough, came home, he's had severe headaches every day since that day. Because his mind remembers the headache. Jason remembers. He remembers every fact. Play Jeopardy with him—he's amazing." In this account, which reproduces Dr. Novak's explanatory model with remarkable acuity, an analogical relation is drawn between remembering facts and remembering pain. Jason's brain *remembered* pain because "that's how his brain is wired," as Debbie later put it.

As Debbie's comments suggest, Jason was a high-achieving student who performed at the top of his honors and AP classes in his public high school in spite of his struggles with pain. Over the years, he had tried numerous medications, even though they often brought side effects worse than the original symptoms. His family also made a sustained commitment to complementary and alternative therapies, including physical therapy, hypnotherapy, acupuncture, Pilates, and yoga. This was not always easy, because, as Debbie pointed out, the therapies were not convenient for patients who attended school regularly. She lamented of Meg Pratt: "She wanted to see him twice a week during the week. And she works between nine and five. Well, I have a kid who wants to go to school full-time." The fact that Meg's office took almost an hour to get to during the afternoon rush hour made it even more difficult to fit in appointments.

Debbie reported spending hundreds of dollars per week on Jason's co-pays. Her two older children were out of college but still in need of financial support (with one unemployed and living at home), and they sometimes resented the fact that their parents appeared to have more money to spend on Jason. Meanwhile, the family business had suffered in the recent recession. "My husband's work is crap, you know," Debbie told me. "No one's making money." Certainly, few people were spending money on high-end interior design, the focus of Debbie's husband's business.

Like many West Clinic patients, Jason was somewhat suspicious of treatments that he viewed as psychological. "I want to see, like, things that are actually concrete like medicine, or doing something. I don't believe in like, doing mental things. . . . I don't like when people sort of hint that this is all in my head, and that I can control it. 'Cause I think this is a real problem." When I interviewed him, he had just begun seeing Donna Buckley, a psychologist who had joined the West Clinic team relatively recently. When I asked what kinds of things they were working on, he responded, "Like, things with your thoughts, you know, changing your thoughts, relaxation, stuff like that." Because of what he termed Donna's "scientific" approach, Jason did not call this therapy.

Although Jason was similar to many of the adolescents that I encountered in the West Clinic, he stood out to me because of the stark mismatch between the clinic's explanatory framework and his family's own understanding of certain aspects of his pain. Early on, Debbie told me, Rebecca Hunter had written in her report that Jason had Asperger syndrome. "Why?" Debbie asked, in recounting this story, her voice crackling with anger. "Because Jason came in and he said, 'You know, I really don't have friends.' Listen to what he said: 'I don't have friends because I was in a wheelchair for two years and my friends, after a while, dumped me. They didn't have time for me.' This is not a child that cannot make friends. In the classroom, he thrived. He had a million friends in the classroom. Outside, nobody wants to wheel an eleven-year-old around." Here, Debbie raised an alternative explanation for her son's social troubles: his lack of friends was situational and should not be interpreted as evidence of an underlying social dysfunction. What evolved the following year appeared to support Debbie's explanation. Jason got out of his wheelchair, and, at Rebecca's behest, made it a point to make friends. Soon, Rebecca determined that Jason was functioning much better and said that she no longer needed to see the Katz family.

Jason's case was not unique with respect to the rift that emerged between clinical and familial explanations. In many ways, in fact, his case was similar to that of Mark Siegel, whose family resisted the suggestion that his pain was intractable because his brain was "sticky." The two boys, both Jewish, even lived in the same community and their mothers had spoken on the phone and traded notes regarding their sons' pain. Like Julie Siegel, Debbie Katz had an outspoken personality and was driven by an overriding sense of injustice with respect to her son's suffering, characteristics that had contributed to both women being labeled by the pain team as "pushy."[17] But what made Jason's case stand apart was that, by the time that I met him at least, he did not seem to exhibit any of the qualities of PDD. His affect was certainly flat when I saw him in the clinic, but I attributed this more to his frustrations with long clinic wait times and dead-end treatments than I did to an underlying emotional processing problem. However, while Rebecca Hunter had moved on, Dr. Petrosian was still suggesting that Jason's brain was "sticky."

I first met Jason during my first summer of fieldwork, when he visited the West Clinic for frequent appointments with Dr. Petrosian while Dr. Novak, his previous physician, was away on vacation. I sat in on Jason's first appointment with Dr. Petrosian and listened to Debbie explain, with a strong note of urgency in her voice, how Jason had been suffering for five years, how she had promised him that they would get rid of his pain by his bar mitzvah, and now simply hoped that he would be able to go to college in a few years. Debbie seemed exhausted, and Jason seemed angry.

During one of these early visits, I had a revealing conversation with a nurse who was working in the clinic at the time. The nurse made an offhand comment about the strangeness of the Katz family. When I responded that I didn't think that the family seemed strange, that I had sympathy for Debbie and understood why she felt so frustrated, the nurse looked at me long and hard for several seconds and then repeated that she really did think it was a strange family. Feeling a bit put on the spot, I suggested that perhaps they were too much like other families I knew for me to have noticed this quality. She mentioned the high degree of stress and pressure, and I simply nodded my head.

Later that fall, Dr. Petrosian told Jason that he needed to make some lifestyle changes because he had too much going on and was working too hard; his body was paying the price. I had heard this logic before, but something did not square for me with Dr. Petrosian's analysis. It was certainly true that Jason was staying up until 1 A.M. during the school year because he had five hours of homework each night for his AP classes, but he also spent several hours in the early evening talking to his friends online, which seemed to me a healthy dose of leisure. Jason's life was not hyperscheduled to the extent that Lila Feldman's had been; in fact, he had foregone participation in most extracurricular activities because his weekday afternoons had for so long been occupied with various CAM therapies. While Dr. Petrosian's warnings rang true for West Clinic patients in general, they did not seem the most applicable to Jason's particular case.

Jason, for his part, denied that lack of sleep and academic stress made his pain worse. He pointed out to Dr. Petrosian that his pain had been worse over the summer, even though he had worked *less* and slept more. "If anything," Jason told me, "my pain sometimes gets worse over the summer 'cause I have nothing to do. When I'm distracted, it gets a little better." Repeated admonishments to take fewer AP classes made little sense to Jason, because he enjoyed them and did not feel that they created stress.

Moreover, whereas patients like Brittany Rogers admitted to feeling an incredible amount of pressure to perform every academic detail perfectly, Jason maintained that he did the bare minimum necessary to get an A. Debbie explained, "He doesn't go above and beyond. He doesn't go crazy studying. He knows how to get the A's, you know. And that's why, you know, people are, 'Oh, you're so stressed this must be stress.' And he's like, 'Well, I'm really not stressed. You're making me stressed.'" Debbie laughed, and then continued, "And that's why they think that he should go see a therapist. He's like, 'I'm really not stressed. I know I'm gonna get the A's. I know I'll get into a college. I'm not stressed about it.'" When Jason and Debbie tried to insist that Jason was not stressed, however, they were typically told that he must be unaware of it, because he was carrying his stress inside his body.

From my perspective, it sounded as if Jason's clinicians were trying to put him into a box that was not a clear fit. As I have discussed elsewhere in this book, diagnostic typecasting can give way to misrecognition. The "stressed out" adolescent is a familiar cultural and clinical trope, yet it seemed in this case that Jason was being stretched to fit this mold and, in the process, distorted. At the same time, the sharp difference between my own reaction to Jason's family and that of the West Clinic nurse should remind us how much the interpretation of meaning is shaped by social position. To me, Jason Katz did not seem strange, in part, perhaps, because he came from a family background similar to my own: Jewish, upper-middle-class, and achievement-oriented. Similarly, clinical (mis)readings of stress depend on value-laden judgments about work, time, and everyday habits. While Jason's case illustrates the perils of accepting received cultural narratives, such as the one linking pain to adolescent stress, it also highlights the potential blind spots of ethnographers as analysts.

The anthropologist Junko Kitanaka suggests that causal narratives about the relationship between overwork, on the one hand, and depression and suicide, on the other, can provide a "cover story" for more complex explanations.[18] Such narratives also leave unanswered crucial questions about how we assign blame—chiefly, should blame be placed at the level of society for fostering conditions that favor social suffering? Or with the individual whose personality drives them to such behavior?

## THE SICK ADOLESCENT IN SOCIETY

One of the enduring insights of Talcott Parsons's notion of the sick role is that illness entails a social contract between the person and society. The concept highlights the fundamental tension between the person accommodating society's unruly demands, and society accommodating the person's illness, which poses its own challenges for the maintenance of the social and moral order. Several West Clinic therapists lamented, for example, that American schools do not do more to take care of children with chronic illness. While most schools recognized the physical limitations that accompany chronic pain and permitted children to use elevators that were typically off-limits, many were less flexible about the ramifications of extended absences. An important sticking point for

Rebecca Hunter, who devoted many hours of uncompensated work to contacting patients' schools and advocating for specific accommodations, was that adolescents should be permitted to restore their social activities even if academic activities were lagging. Therefore, she often argued that children should go back to school for lunch even before they were ready to make a full return to classes.

The expectation that schools should adjust their policies to cater to chronically ill students reflects an underlying culture of individualism in which middle-class Americans have come to feel entitled to have their children recognized, in institutional settings, as unique individuals with particular preferences, values, habits, and needs. The rise of "individualized education programs" for students with intellectual disabilities and other special needs in recent years shows that the educational infrastructure has been willing to meet such demands. That such accommodations were less readily available to West Clinic patients may reflect a deeply entrenched ambivalence about chronic pain in American society. If Jon Morgan was correct in observing that his son's school was much more accommodating of a student who broke her arm around the same time that Zack developed CRPS, this differential treatment may result from the stigma surrounding illnesses that seem traceable to a psychological cause. The inflexibility of schools with respect to chronic pain was one reason why a significant number of West Clinic patients (almost half of those who I interviewed) ended up temporarily withdrawing from school. The struggle for accommodations had made such a profound impression on seventeen-year-old Melinda Worthington—who had difficulty taking her own notes due to pain in her hands, yet was accused of laziness when she tried to get out of writing—that it had shaped her future aspirations and desire to study public policy.

Patients like Brittany Rogers and Jason Katz, who maintained their regular academic schedules with little interruption, were usually viewed as less serious cases than patients who withdrew from school. If a patient attended school regularly, he or she was typically judged to be "functioning," a psychological label that masks the often-debilitating effects of life with chronic pain. In this way, acclimating to long-standing pain had the unfortunate effect of downplaying the severity of symptoms in relation to therapeutic goals. As Debbie Katz put it, in a creative twist on this clinical language, "Don't tell me that we think your kid's better because he can *function*. Because he goes to school and he's getting good grades. That doesn't mean my kid is 'functioning.' That doesn't mean he's better."

Furthermore, the fact that some clinicians only scheduled appointments during normal school hours was a source of tension for the parents of patients who were ostensibly "functioning." Anne Rothschild mused, "You know, you guys tell us to treat 'em like normal kids, . . . not force 'em, but send 'em off to school, don't pick 'em up from school. . . . but then you're saying, you gotta see this therapist, this therapist, you know, and do all this to get them better." As Anne's comments imply, regularly missing school for health-care appointments undercuts the logic of normalization that aimed to restore adolescents to their preexisting social roles.

For patients like Lila Feldman and Eli Lerner, however, the sick role offered a clear if somewhat precarious respite from the normal stresses of adolescent life. Whenever illness appears as a means to a potentially desirable end, even if ambivalently so, it raises important questions about agency. In a brief yet provocative essay written several decades ago, the anthropologists Nancy Scheper-Hughes and Margaret Lock suggested that Parsons's concept of the sick role offers a useful template for thinking about illness as an occasion of resistance.[19] Assuming the sick role, Scheper-Hughes and Lock argue, signifies, among other things, a refusal: to work, to go to school, to care for one's loved ones.[20] Although this reading distorts Parsons's functionalist emphasis on restoring social harmony, it is nevertheless helpful for demonstrating the tactical ends that illness may achieve.

Over my time in the West Clinic, there were other subtle signs of this logic of refusal. Earlier in this chapter, I mentioned the patient whom the pain team believed was "holding on" to her pain to avoid playing sports at the collegiate level. Similarly, Charlotte LeFevre suggested at another team meeting that an injury sustained by a docile male patient offered a means to escape having to play football. In Lila Feldman's case, the exemptions afforded by chronic pain opened her eyes to the risky personal calculus of predicating all of her future happiness on her acceptance to Stanford, and even Brittany Rogers admitted that she was happy to take a break from her taxing dance schedule. Insofar as these illness episodes lent themselves to a broader form of social critique, they may also be seen as subtly orchestrated acts of refusal.

This logic of refusal figures the body as a key source of power—potentially the only one available to adolescents. A former West Clinic therapist with whom I spoke noted, "The kids have no power but their bodies sometimes. So you'll find that consciously or unconsciously that's a way to get power. Because a sick kid, people have to be nice to. Can't ignore them." This incisive social commentary on the category of the child nicely demonstrates a more general set of anthropological observations about modes of embodied resistance among poor, marginalized, or otherwise vulnerable people.[21] It highlights, more specifically, the limited means of middle-class American youth to resist parental or societal demands. Middle-class Americans have adopted an ambivalent cultural model of adolescent autonomy that conceptualizes adolescents' dependency as both problematic and necessary. The logic of embodied refusal offers one way of understanding how adolescents resist such contradictory expectations while giving the appearance of compliance.

The difficulty with framing pain in terms of refusal, however, is that, particularly in light of the morally loaded history of psychosomatic medicine, such readings of patient agency might appear to suggest that symptoms are fabricated. In this way, understanding pain as a form of resistance can imply that it is unreal or inauthentic and, in so doing, delegitimize it.[22] There is thus a politics of recognition at stake in judgments about social sources of suffering.

Because American culture privileges youth as especially deserving of special protections, their status provides a good beacon of societal well-being during periods of social breakdown. Consider the recent outbreak of a mysterious disorder in Le Roy, New York, characterized by twitching, tics, and verbal outbursts, and primarily affecting adolescent girls. While multiple etiological theories were postulated, including environmental exposures and mass conversion disorder, many observers ultimately linked the strange disorder to the steep economic decline of this working-class community.[23] Such theories propose that youth embody the effects of broader social and economic vulnerability, suggesting that much more is at stake in these illnesses than an individual ailing body.

When standard biomedical frameworks fail to offer convincing explanatory narratives, patients, clinicians, and society at large turn to alternative interpretive resources for making sense of illness. This chapter has probed what biomedical explanatory frameworks may otherwise occlude—that is, the broader forms of social unrest that give shape to the embodiment of stress. More than the explanatory frameworks explored in previous chapters, this strand of explanatory theorizing specifically highlights the limits of clinical interventions for curing pediatric pain. While the West Clinic staff enjoyed some success intervening in family systems, it was much more difficult for them to effect meaningful, durable changes in schools or larger institutional structures. This also helps to explain why these explanatory narratives were particularly appealing to clinicians in the interview arena: they absolved clinicians from taking responsibility for the limits—and failures—of clinical intervention.

The cases explored in this chapter likewise highlight the classed dimensions of patienthood and the chronic pain experience, showing that causal narratives of illness are shaped by specific class positions and temporal conditions. Beginning with George Beard's notion of "American nervousness," psychosomatic illnesses in the United States have revealed cultural preoccupations with the mental and physical tolls of socioeconomic privilege. From this perspective, the discourse on stress—and specifically, its relationship to (ill) health—encodes specific moral judgments about work and activity.[24] In this way, stress may become what Emily Martin has called an "object of desire," insofar as it interlaces with cultural models of, and aspirations for, success and productivity. However, as Martin also points out, illnesses are never stable objects of cultural desire; they also convey the anxieties of losing one's grip on one's body, which may come to stand as a metaphor for larger forms of social and economic control.[25]

Although Lila Feldman, Eli Lerner, and Jason Katz all faced stress with respect to their college prospects, their anxieties took shape in markedly different ways. Eli's case, in particular, highlights the embodied effects of economic precarity, illustrating how pain articulates with broader forms of social dislocation. In doing so, it painfully demonstrates the limits of the West Clinic's therapeutic approach for families that were struggling financially.

Furthermore, as Jason Katz's story reminds us, not all families accepted the persuasive power of the explanatory link between adolescent stress and pain. While anthropologists have for decades argued for increased attention to the social relations of sickness, it is important to remember that the pendulum may swing too far in this direction. Less often recognized in anthropological work are the subtle ways in which arguments about social causality may gloss over the rich complexities, layers, and ambivalences of individual cases, and, in doing so, misidentify disparate sources of suffering.[26] Attention to social frames should not, therefore, eclipse the personal, particular, and moral dimensions of individual illness.

It is in this spirit that I have resisted totalizing narratives that link outcomes and responses to specific explanatory variables. It bears mentioning here that Lila Feldman, Eli Lerner, and Jason Katz all hailed from Jewish families, yet their Jewishness did not necessarily play a role in how they experienced the link between pain and stress. Stress filters into families in different ways, which may or may not have anything to do with ethnicity.

This chapter has thus highlighted the multiplicity and contingency of explanatory frames for illness. Stress rarely constitutes a singular illness agent. Instead, it is woven into complex accounts of illness, within which it tends to stand in for a larger sense of ambiguity, uncertainty, or irresolution. It is no accident, then, that in charting the role of stress in the illness experience of West Clinic patients, I have looped back to explanatory frames visited earlier in this book, such as personality and pathological family ties. What these cases make clear is that explanatory frames serve as interpretive resources that people may draw on piecemeal for different reasons, at different points in the therapeutic trajectory. Recognition of stress may help families assign meaning to the experience of chronic pain without it being labeled a proximate cause of illness.

Brittany Rogers is a useful case in point. Although Brittany and her mother, Jane, responded positively to the stress hypothesis, the last link in their chain of causal reasoning isolated a much more specific biomechanical cause. For this, they credited, not the West Clinic, which they nevertheless praised highly, but an intrepid chiropractor whom Brittany's father had originally consulted. After learning what Brittany was dealing with, the chiropractor urged the Rogers to let her take X-rays of Brittany's spine. Later that week, Jane googled *rectus abdominus*, which she had learned was the name of the muscle that was bothering Brittany. This search sent her to a page from *Gray's Anatomy*. "And I read, oh, the nerve that controls the rectus abdominus comes from T12. And I was like, woah, that's weird," Jane recalled. "So the next day I went to the chiropractor and I said, 'Look, I'm probably not telling you anything you don't know,' and I told her what I did. She says, 'Well, let's look at the X-ray.' And we looked and every—it was like, parallel, parallel, parallel, perfect, and you get to T12 and it was clearly out of whack." The chiropractor adjusted Brittany's twelfth thoracic vertebra, and her relief was immediate. Charlotte and Tess had brought her pain rating down from a "ten" to a six or a seven, but the chiropractor brought it down to a three or a four at most, and some nights Brittany had no pain at all.

I asked Jane whether she had shared this discovery with Dr. Novak or Dr. Sterling, whom Brittany was also seeing at the time. She acknowledged being "a little bit worried because I know some doctors don't like chiropractic." The chiropractor had told her that she had to choose whether she wanted to do "natural or medical," which bothered Jane, whose attitude was to take "the best of both worlds," a perspective that aligned very well with the West Clinic's approach. When it came down to it, Jane told me, "They just said, 'Yeah, good for you.' So that's all they said, you know. I mean, they want the kid to get better."

Brittany's case was somewhat unusual, insofar as her family was eventually able to pinpoint a specific cause for her pain with a great deal of certainty. Far more typical, however, was their cycling through a number of different explanatory frames: Dr. Novak's initial neurobiological reading, concerns about family dynamics, and the high level of stress on adolescents in middle-class American society. Although the explanation that the Rogers family finally adopted was quite straightforward, this simple biomechanical account belies the multilayered progression of explanatory reasoning that I have traced through the pages of this book. It is precisely such interpretive reasoning that lies at the core of chronic pain experience.

# Conclusion

One night in December, several months after I had formally completed my data collection, I drove across town to visit the Harris family. I had left several messages on their answering machine over the preceding few months, and when I finally reached Kay on her cell phone, she apologized profusely for her delay in responding. Things had been especially hectic since the new school year started, because Rob, her husband, had just gone back to school. The next evening, at Kay's suggestion, I ventured out to their home, hoping that a final meeting would provide a sense of closure for their participation in the study.

When I arrived, Michael met me at the front door, the fragrant smell of freshly baked cookies wafting in from the kitchen. "You have to taste one and make sure they're okay," Kay urged as I appeared in the doorway. I helped myself to a warm chocolate chip cookie and asked how things were going. I knew that Michael had begun the school year at a new middle school because of the bullying problem the previous year. I was eager to hear how the transition, which had been a major focus of his therapy in the West Clinic, was going. Michael told me that he had almost no pain, but that he was still dealing with some anxiety. Kay added that school was "still an issue," but that Michael had "come a really far way."

Together, Kay and Michael filled me in on Michael's rocky start. During his first few days at his new school, he had been crippled by overwhelming anxiety. The bus rides were torturous, not because of his new classmates, but because of his own flood of distressing emotion. Each day, he would send despondent text messages to his parents during the ride to school. By 9 A.M., he would call Kay in tears, begging to be picked up. In the beginning, Kay had obliged Michael's requests, not knowing what else to do. Finally, however, the assistant principal intervened. On one morning when Michael went to the office to call his mother, as had become his routine, the assistant principal told Michael that he could not go home. Michael threatened to call the police and to say that he was being held against his will, and the assistant principal, unfazed, responded that it was illegal for Michael to stay home and not go to school, and that *he* would be the one to get in trouble should he call the police. This turning of the tables only incensed Michael further.

But then something happened. The assistant principal tried a different tack. He confessed that he, too, had suffered from anxiety, and said he understood what Michael was going through. He did not care if Michael sat in his office the whole day, but he was going to stay at school, and they would get through it together. And they did. The assistant principal sat with Michael, and talked to him, and Michael eventually went back to his classes. He still struggled with his anxiety and he still dreaded the bus ride to school, but he had come a long way over the course of the year since he had stopped attending school. When I last saw him that December evening, the road ahead was uncertain, but by all accounts, he seemed to be doing okay.

This temporary ending to Michael's story was typical of those that I encountered during my time in the West Clinic. Few adolescents appeared to make a complete recovery, and many struggled with emotional distress even if the pain faded away. Most patients, however, seemed to do better over the course of their treatment. When I asked the pain team in interviews about how the West Clinic patients responded, most said that patients typically got better *if* they invested in treatment. Admittedly, this is a big "if," one that lets clinicians off the hook for therapeutic failures. And, of course, my research demonstrates that there were important exceptions to this rule. Jason Katz, for example, made a serious commitment to multidisciplinary therapies but got worse over the course of his treatment. Nevertheless, the basic thrust of this assessment—that most, though not all, patients experienced some benefit from treatment if they stuck around long enough—aligned with my own observations in the West Clinic.

What this improvement looked like on the ground varied quite a bit, however. Charlotte LeFevre estimated that 90 percent of the patients she worked with showed some improvement, and 50 to 60 percent had remained pain-free ever since. She told a particularly poignant story concerning a high-school senior with CRPS whose therapeutic goal had been to attend her senior prom. One day, the patient, who had been using a wheelchair and then a walker, simply stood up at the end of her session and walked into the other room, as if she had forgotten all about the intense pain from walking. "So this was real, there wasn't any deal with this," Charlotte said, to assure me that the patient hadn't been faking. "Her mother turned around and both of us started to cry. You know, I mean, 'cause it was such a huge thing. That was probably one of the most, of course, amazing dynamic experiences." I asked whether the patient had gone to her prom. "Of course," Charlotte gushed, eager to share the story. "Actually, it was amazing. I hadn't spoken to her in months, and I just sometimes will check. I called and her mom said, 'Hold on one second.' She came running to the phone and she said, 'I can't believe you're calling now. I was going to call and I totally forgot. I'm on my way to the prom.' It was like there was some connection with that. Oh my god, it was just—'Oh don't talk to me; just go.' She said, 'No, I wanted to, and I'm wearing the blue dress.'"

While Charlotte's story was remarkable for the dramatic recovery and auspiciously timed phone call, few clinicians were as optimistic about their patients' recovery. Tess Bergman, the yoga instructor, noted, "I think that they do get better but they don't get as better as I would want them. . . . I think that my definition of better is a little different than it used to be." The physical therapist Meg Pratt offered a similarly subdued assessment: "I think the problem is that they still have those-whatever it is that caused them to start having the [pain]—you know, the pressure from parents or the dysfunction in the family, is still going on. So they learn better tools to deal with it, but I think they still are gonna have—most of them have residuals afterwards." Such statements convey both a pragmatic orientation toward therapeutic success and a subtle hint of disappointment that their work did not have more enduring effects.

Among the most modest estimates of improvement were those from Ted Bridgewater and Craig Davies, who reported that 50 percent and 25 percent of their patients, respectively, experienced a significant reduction in pain. This may be because their treatment modalities, acupuncture and craniosacral therapy, were the most passive therapies that the West Clinic offered. In these settings, the patient was merely expected to show up for treatment, and not to learn "tools" or "skills." Consequently, patient "investment"—to use the clinicians' terminology—in these therapeutic encounters meant something quite different than it did for hypnotherapy, physical therapy, or yoga. This suggests that to invest in one's treatment in a way that catalyzes therapeutic benefits means to invest as an *active* patient.

This is not to say that patients were necessarily assigned an unfair burden of responsibility in arbitrations of therapeutic efficacy. Such views have been popularized in recent years by reading ideologies of self-care through neoliberal logics of self-governance, which suggest that health care has increasingly fallen to patients and their families in the wake of global shifts in political economy that divest states of such responsibility. However, I join a growing number of scholars who have expressed skepticism about automatically subsuming a clinical emphasis on responsibility and self-care under the label of neoliberalism.[1] Instead, I find a persuasive alternative in Annemarie Mol's 2008 book, *The Logic of Care: Health and the Problem of Patient Choice.* In this much-acclaimed work, Mol illustrates that care can sometimes be enhanced when professionals supply less "product" and patients do more work themselves. In a similar way, I have come to view the emphasis on self-care exhibited by the West Clinic's therapeutic ideologies as a productive and generative component of pain management that was not always (or not necessarily) accompanied by a default of clinical responsibility. For Michael Harris, for example, therapeutic progress hinged on his successful use of hypnotherapy, yet he learned and exercised these skills in the context of his relationship with Charlotte LeFevre, who was clearly very invested in his treatment.

Mol notes that we tend to think of medical care as either something that is provided by practitioners to a submissive patient, or something that patients do for themselves in an individualizing, neoliberal mode. Yet there is an important sense in which care is more collaborative and interactive than in this simplified view, which risks obscuring the relational dynamics of treatment. In other words, modes of self-care may create responsibilities for the patient, and yet do so within a social milieu, in the context of caring, committed therapeutic relationships.

If we return to Julie Livingston's notion of the clinic as a microcosm,[2] the possibilities that I take away from this clinical ethnography are, first, that care constitutes an important component of pain management that works to disrupt the loneliness of pain, and second, that the creative use of language is a critical resource for making sense of and responding to pain. Yet if these are therapeutic possibilities, then they are so within a particular sociocultural and historical context, and one that is not equally accessible to all American adolescents and their families. Consequently, this book also maps a particular set of relations among culture, care, and economy. The West Clinic and the possibilities it affords bring into critical relief the vulnerabilities and modes of exclusion that structure life outside of it. In this sense, the West Clinic is an exceptional space and not representative of U.S. health care more generally.

## PAIN MANAGEMENT AS RELATIONAL CARE

That Charlotte LeFevre reported higher ratings of therapeutic efficacy than did Ted Bridgewater or Craig Davies suggests to me that, to the extent that pain management is social, it depends on a particular kind of relational care. Charlotte's success as a clinician resulted in large measure from her ability to establish a unique sort of intimacy with her patients. Her gentle demeanor and soothing voice had a calming effect that facilitated an easy rapport with her young patients. It further helped that she saw patients in her living room, which was tastefully decorated in muted shades of yellow and blue. This tranquil environment, combined with Charlotte's warm, empathic persona, did much to instill trust into her patients and led Charlotte to play a major role in the therapeutic successes of patients like Michael Harris, Claire Joffe, Brittany Rogers, and Lila Feldman.

Charlotte's intimate engagement with patients' lives and stories cuts to the core of what this book has been about. One of its central goals has been to illustrate that pain is much more social than we often assume. In drawing attention to the social dimensions of pain experience, I do not mean to discount the ways in which living with chronic pain can be intensely lonely and alienating. As Elaine Scarry has noted, "[Pain] brings with it all the solitude of absolute privacy with none of its safety, all the self-exposure of the utterly public with none of its possibility for camaraderie or shared experience."[3] Nevertheless, in living with, responding to, and interpreting pain, we cannot escape the fact that pain is experienced and understood in worlds that are fundamentally social.

Throughout this book, I have used the concepts of "onstage" and "backstage" clinical spaces as metaphors for thinking about how the clinic intersects with broader arenas of human social life and dimensions of public and private. While Erving Goffman's dramaturgical approach to social interaction was designed to convey the performative nature of everyday life, it is particularly well suited to thinking about the sociality of pain. In a paradoxical way, without visual evidence of their pain, chronic pain patients must perform the role of the suffering subject to convince others that they are truly in pain, even as this performance calls the reality of their pain into question. In this sense, they are inescapably "onstage" in ways that may threaten to undermine their legitimacy. To care for the person in pain is to temporarily suspend judgment, doubt, and uncertainty in the service of trust and empathy. In this way, observing the social life of pain within and beyond the clinic can tell us a lot about human social interaction more generally—about how we attend to and care for others in their moments of vulnerability.

For West Clinic parents, as for the staff, an emotional commitment to support children's suffering was a critical component of care. Less often acknowledged by the clinicians, however, were the material resources that enabled and sustained such relations of care. In addition to expecting that patients invest actively in therapy, treatment in the West Clinic entailed staggering investments of families' time and money—investments of a kind that, it bears repeating, are simply not an option for many American families. Each appointment kept and paid for, each day off from work, each vacation forestalled, and each bit of time and attention diverted from a patient's healthy sibling reflected a powerful (and privileged) commitment by parents to acknowledge and relieve their children's pain.

Parents were evaluated on the basis of these commitments and criticized when appointments were dropped or telephone calls not made. This underscores that parents are always "onstage" in such institutional encounters, exposed to the penetrating gaze of professional judgment.[4] Just as their adolescent children were forced to perform their pain or risk having it denied, parents, once enrolled in the clinic, had to perform their care in material and affective ways or have their motives questioned. And, as we saw in chapter 4, they could also go too far in this direction, opening themselves up to the criticism that they could be "caring too much."

In tracking these social dimensions of pain management, this book joins a growing body of work in medical anthropology committed to illuminating the relational dynamics of experiences that are often understood to be intensely private, such as heroin addiction, psychiatric institutionalization, and dying of cancer.[5] A relational lens on suffering exposes the ways in which we are all, even in our moments of greatest solitude, unavoidably shaped by our dependence on others. An underlying message of these works is thus that care for the other is a fundamentally moral enterprise that follows from and overflows the alienation of pain.[6]

Care is deeply situated within ongoing social practice, which is one reason why it has been such an attractive site for recent anthropological inquiry.[7] For all the anthropological attention to care, however, few recent ethnographies of care have focused on adolescents and their distinct vulnerabilities.[8] The West Clinic constitutes a particularly useful case for illustrating the juxtaposition of pain with care, because its patients necessarily begin from a position of social dependency. As such, pain management, for these patients, was always already embedded in existing relations of care. From this perspective, it is not surprising that therapeutic practices often took patients and families beyond medicine and the clinic, and even occasionally seemed to move beyond the pain itself.

Returning to Michael Harris, I have come to view the assistant principal's willingness to sit with Michael and ride out his anxiety as an important form of care that mirrors—and complements—the therapeutic work performed by the pain team. One of the greatest benefits of the West Clinic was the opportunity for patients to be surrounded by caring others. As Mimi Feldman put it, "The best benefit of the pain program, I thought, was that she was surrounded by smart, professional, caring people, who understood that she had this pain problem." This being-together helped patients to overcome the existential isolation and immense vulnerability of pain and, sometimes, of adolescence itself. Many patients had been so debilitated by pain that they had given up nearly all of their old routines and activities. In their place, the pain program provided a structure for everyday living. The clinicians, in turn, offered a temporary safety net, a social scaffold to protect them from the multiple sources of stress in adolescents' social worlds that tend to complicate recovery.

Of course, nurturing relationships did not replace the West Clinic's primary goal of relieving and managing chronic pain, nor were all of the West Clinic families entirely satisfied with this therapeutic by-product. Some families, like the Siegels, did not invest in treatment long enough to develop intimate clinical relationships. Others, like the Katzes, invested in long-term relationships but were profoundly disappointed by the lack of improvement in pain symptoms. In these cases, differing notions of clinical "success" were felt most acutely. Yet crucially, very few families who committed to the program felt abandoned in the ways that they had experienced before coming to the West Clinic.[9]

This extraordinary clinical care also implied a potential limitation, however, for I often wondered how patients who had withdrawn from their normal activities would do once they reentered the world beyond pain. I worried about whether this care would sustain adolescents once they reintegrated into school, sports, and activities with friends. Would the shark's tooth talisman that Charlotte LeFevre had given Michael actually get him through another bullying episode?[10] How would Claire Joffe respond to inappropriate text messages from an older male friend without Tess Bergman there to guide her? In short, what would happen once the clinicians were no longer fixtures in these adolescents' lives? To what extent would their therapeutic efficacy endure? While these questions still trouble me, Michael's story showed me that care can emerge in the unlikeliest of places—even between a figure of disciplinary authority like a middle-school assistant principal and an impetuous thirteen-year-old boy.

Such possibilities for care ultimately return me to the question of pain's sharability with which I started this book. If, as I have suggested, the moral stakes of "sharing pain" point to the obligation of responding to another's suffering, then acknowledging pain through caring for a person in pain is a fundamentally social act that diminishes the isolation of pain.[11] Care and acknowledgment are crucial responses to pain that routinely unfold in both mundane and extraordinary ways. This, I believe, provides reason enough to locate pain, not only in some private vacuum of interiority but also in what the anthropologist Michael Jackson has called the "in-between spaces of intersubjectivity."[12]

## EXPLANATORY FORCE AND CONTINGENCY

This book has adopted language and explanation as fundamental lenses on the social dimensions of pain, suggesting that clinical speech is a particular mode of exercising and articulating care in the clinic. Specifically, it has examined a set of explanatory frameworks—neurobiological, psychodynamic, and societal stress—that clinicians, patients, and families draw on to make sense of pediatric pain, in which "making sense" refers to a collective endeavor of jointly produced meaning. In tracing a series of overlapping explanatory pathways, I have argued that explanations of pain are seldom absolute or monolithic, but rather vary over time and across contexts in addressing evolving interpretive needs.

The notion of backstage and onstage explanatory models highlights the fact that clinicians emphasize different explanatory factors in conversations with patients and families than they do in private clinical spaces. A central contention of this book has been that clinical explanations are designed to persuade patients and families of understandings of pain that will lay the groundwork for certain therapeutic strategies. In the book's first two chapters, I illustrated how pediatric pain clinicians employed neurobiological metaphors and explanatory models of pain when explaining pain to patients and families as a way of legitimizing their pain experience and thwarted attempts to secure effective medical treatment. Particularly in their initial conversations, clinicians often displayed an intuitive sense of what families would be prepared to hear, and what might be inappropriate or even harmful to say in that context.[13] In chapters 3 and 4, however, I showed how, during team meetings, etiological theories more readily embraced discourses of psychological and family blame.

The interviews that I conducted with pediatric pain clinicians constitute another important discursive arena for airing explanations of pain. In this setting, the audience was an inquisitive anthropologist rather than people with a personal stake in pediatric pain. Chapter 5 revealed that explanatory accounts that explicitly linked pain to societal stress were most likely to crop up in these interviews with clinicians. Outside the clinic, the focus of blame more easily shifted beyond the targets of clinical interventions, which tend to focus on individualistic or interpersonal causes. This shift also reflects the difference between talking about pain in general and talking about biographical particulars.

Backstage and onstage clinical spaces and the anthropological interview constitute distinct discourse contexts replete with their own vocabularies, metaphors, and styles of reasoning. This is not to say that discourse contexts were determinative of explanations of pain, or that clinicians did not retain some ambivalence about the very prospect of identifying an underlying cause. Indeed, I have argued from the beginning that chronic pain is characterized by causal multiplicity and a great deal of uncertainty. Nor do I mean to suggest that explanations are always given for purely pragmatic reasons.[14] Nevertheless, insofar as ethnography can help us to see how distinctive voices are differently and contextually deployed across discursive arenas, ethnographic methods are particularly well suited to capturing multiple explanatory discourses. In doing so, they can help us understand how clinicians express and promote competing accounts without observers, or the clinicians themselves, necessarily viewing them as incongruities.

Still, if my sustained attention to the rhetorical dimensions of clinical explanations has brought to light how multiple explanatory frameworks can operate together, readers may be left with lingering questions about how some of these explanatory frames relate to clinicians' underlying understandings of pain and the world. How do these explanations accord with clinicians' actual beliefs about pain?[15] To what extent is talk of "smart neurons" and "sticky brains" just rhetoric, and to what extent does it map onto underlying understandings? I have two responses to these questions.

The first is that the clinicians found these to be useful for explaining complex ideas in clear and straightforward ways. Colloquial understandings of smart neurons and sticky brains draw on folk neurobiology in a way that runs parallel to, rather than countering, scientific knowledge. For clinicians, if these metaphors appeared to work in a practical sense, it was because they built on, and borrowed from, scientific models. In this sense, we might think of these concepts as metaphors for a more complex set of relations between memory, attention, neural signaling, and pain. Here, it is also important to keep in mind that the West Clinic's pain team hailed from diverse professional backgrounds with varying levels of exposure to scientific research on pain; we can therefore expect that they varied in the extent to which they regarded these heuristics as accurate representations.

My second response returns me to a point made in chapter 2 about the pragmatics of truth. A pragmatic orientation to truth redirects the line of questioning above to ask about the added value of concepts like smart neurons and sticky brains in terms of explanatory currency. The point, from this perspective, is not whether clinicians believe these concepts are true, but rather what sorts of practical social and therapeutic effects they can enable and produce.

Throughout this book, I have used "all in your head" as a placeholder to capture the uncertainty and stigmatization that often accompany explanatory contingency and explanatory failure. Yet this label, as an explanatory metaphor for pain, does something more than describe a type of pain that is dubious and poorly understood. It also generates a response in the listener, which is not generally positive. This tendency points to the performative function of language and to the philosopher of language John L. Austin's distinction between meaning and force. For Austin, whose work provides an important foundation for viewing language as a form of social action, meaning "is equivalent to the word's sense and reference," while force refers to the action that the word performs when someone utters it.[16] The meaning of the statement "all in your head" might be nothing more than a psychological explanation for pain, but its force, in moral terms, is arguably much greater: it delegitimizes the patient's suffering, denies her humanity, and creates strong affective pulls. Another way of framing the sociality of pain, then, is to say that the words we use to explain it have real effects in the body and in the social world.

The concept of *language ideology* has been central to recent scholarship in linguistic anthropology but has not yet been fully explored by medical anthropologists interested in language.[17] This concept conveys not only that cultural ideologies, or commonsense beliefs and assumptions about the world, are "constituted, encoded, or enacted in language," but also that "notions of how communication works as a social process, and to what purpose, are culturally variable and need to be discovered rather than simply assumed."[18] Some scholars have suggested, with good evidence, that biomedical practitioners subscribe to a referentialist language ideology—that is, the idea that the primary function of language is to represent things sincerely or truthfully rather than to express desires or perform other social functions.[19] Yet sometimes the hegemonic nature of this ideology is assumed rather than demonstrated.[20] This tendency may result, in part, from reducing the language ideologies of biomedicine to those of the natural sciences, even though the practice of clinical medicine is as much an art as a science.[21] Nevertheless, I believe that such ideas depend on a caricaturized view of biomedicine that is worth reconsidering here.

Critical studies of medicine have documented the performative functions of language by illustrating how naming, framing, and labeling disease has important social and material consequences.[22] Many of these works are inspired by the philosopher Ian Hacking's notion of the "looping effects" of human kinds.[23] This theory suggests that labels interact with the people to whom we apply them, such that people change and modify their behavior and self-understandings in response to classificatory schemes. For example, when parents are told that their newborn baby has screened positive for a rare genetic disorder, they may treat this baby as sick even if she never manifests symptoms, which can in turn affect the child's developing sense of self.[24] Similarly, popular discourses surrounding autism as a "neurostructural" disorder have come to shape autistic subjects' self-understanding as being differently "wired."[25]

Even within mainstream biomedicine itself, practitioners have recognized the performative dimensions of language. Physicians' reluctance to name potentially fatal diseases like AIDS and cancer reveals a preoccupation with the devastating power of words.[26] Likewise, recent work in placebo studies has drawn attention to the ways in which calling an inert substance a treatment can have powerful healing effects.[27] The placebo mechanism highlights the pragmatic power of imagination, hope, and therapeutic expectations, all of which are framed in important ways by the strategic use of communication.[28] Moreover, while the use of placebos is well known in randomized controlled trials, physicians' use of placebos in clinical practice may be more common than we assume. In one survey of academic physicians, 45 percent of respondents indicated that they had prescribed a placebo.[29] Such findings reveal that physicians believe, not only in the mind-body connection, but also in the power of words, meanings, and expectations to catalyze physiological changes.[30] They also challenge dominant cultural conceptualizations of physicians as staunch mind-body dualists.

Along with such work, this book points beyond a referential perspective on language and challenges conventional social-scientific critiques of biomedical language ideologies. By demonstrating that rhetoric is a tool of medicine that draws on different discourse genres to demystify, clarify, and make sense of pain, I have illustrated how medical practitioners, as a matter of routine clinical practice, rely on the expressive dimensions of language. This includes, of course, the capacity to facilitate healing through the creative deployment of metaphors, images, and words. As Laurence Kirmayer notes: "Words may be used in many different ways to heal: through magical invocation, supplication, or prayer; through dialogue that brings one into relation with an other, present or imagined; as recipes to follow, sources of instructions and imperatives; as conceptual toolkits, sources of metaphors, analogies, and models to think with; as instruments to focus and occupy consciousness, as in the use of mantras; as objects of aesthetic contemplation, as in lyric poetry, to admire their sound and fit; and as stories to dwell within or labyrinths to explore."[31]

Yet, as I also have shown, the performative nature of language in medicine does not foreclose the possibility that words may obstruct the work of treatment, as when a physician says, "It's all in your head," or claims that a patient has a "sticky brain." This capacity for doctors' words to harm their patients underscores several important points made by linguists regarding language and power more generally: that the performative function of language may not be distributed evenly in society, and that speech can be particularly injurious when it is wielded by people with power against those without it.[32] One of the most important contributions of social scientists to the sociocultural study of medicine has been to delineate how medical authority is wielded, and how this can be accomplished subtly, through language, in addition to more overt mechanisms of social control.[33] In other words, if medicine acts as an agent of power, it does so, not only through large-scale processes, such as the medicalization of children's hyperactive behavior,[34] but also in more subtle, everyday ways, through the clinical operation of discursive power.

What are the implications of moving beyond a referentialist language ideology, moving "beyond the words" in the limited sense of their meaning, for social studies of medicine, and for medical practitioners themselves?[35] Taking seriously the possibility that biomedical practitioners may be aware of the performativity of medical language—that is, the capacity to change bodies and lives through words, metaphors, models, and stories—produces new opportunities for critical analysts of medicine. Specifically, this sort of generous reading of the lives and work of biomedical practitioners can lead to studies that move beyond pure critique to focus on the creative potential of medical discourse. To view the language of medicine from a performative perspective is to imbue it with the generative capacities of social reproduction, which sustains and transforms cultural values and practices over time. In short, positioning language and interaction as tools of medicine maps a new set of relations between language and bodies and offers new ways of theorizing therapeutic effects.

## WHEN EXPLANATIONS REST

One day, a few weeks after her mother's surgery, I offered to pick Claire Joffe up after her yoga class with Tess Bergman and entertain her between therapy appointments. We spent the afternoon window-shopping at the local mall and eating food-court pizza after Claire, in a moment of keen resonance with the ethnographic enterprise, proposed that she would teach me "how to be a teenager." After missing almost an entire school year due to her illness, her newfound interest in the mall (she had had little time for shopping when she was busy with sports) had helped Claire to restore some sense of normalcy and reengage with her peers. On this hot summer day, I was happy to oblige.

Later, I drove Claire to Rebecca Hunter's office, where she was meeting her parents and sister for family therapy. During the short drive across town from the mall to Rebecca's office, Claire asked me if I had gotten everything that I "needed" from our time together. "We didn't really talk too much about *that* stuff," she said. I paused, somewhat discomfited by the shift in frame produced by Claire's keying into the transactional nature of our relationship after a pleasant afternoon at the mall. After thinking for a moment, I asked if she thought that her seizures had abated since the initial dip following the news of her mother's surgery. She thought they had, somewhat. I also asked if she was in any pain at all. She shook her head no.

"It's all in my head now," she said. "So I need to work on that."

I wondered aloud what Claire had meant by that. The lingering "it" suggested that there was more to Claire's illness, from her perspective, than the presence or absence of pain. She replied that everyone, all of the doctors, knew that there was nothing physically wrong with her. Somewhat unsettled by this response, I tried to change the subject, and asked which medications she was taking. She told me that she was still taking two Lexapro, and then asked if this was a "real" pill. I said that it was, and asked why she had asked me that. She responded that she knew that sometimes doctors gave "crazy people" fake pills. "Do you think you're crazy?" I asked. "Yes," she said. "Isn't that clear?" She knew everyone thought that she should just get over this and get on with it, and that's what she needed to do.

After six months of treatment in the West Clinic, I was somewhat taken aback that this was where Claire's causal reasoning had landed: "all in my head" and "crazy." I wavered over whether to accept her self-assessments at face value or to try to persuade her that she wasn't crazy. After a moment's hesitation, I chose the latter route, using a strategy that I had often heard used in the West Clinic: it was "all in her head" to the extent that her neurons were located in her brain. To my own ears, however, my effort sounded feeble, and I doubted that Claire put much stock in my response. After months of Dr. Novak maintaining that some unknown event was "eating" Claire inside, it was somewhat difficult to dispute this logic.

In a thoughtful essay from which this section heading is borrowed, the anthropologist Joseph Dumit observes, following the philosopher Ludwig Wittgenstein, that "explanations come to an end somewhere."[36] In stating this self-evident claim, Dumit draws attention to the unsettled, temporary, and local nature of some forms of medical explanation, suggesting that some explanations end, not because meaning is saturated, but because the interpretation is, in his words, "good enough."

For West Clinic patients, explanations came to an end somewhere, whether or not the pain remained. Sometimes, as with Claire Joffe, this end did not seem very distant from where they began. Yet some, like Michael Harris, were able to situate their pain in a new language game, to use Wittgenstein's term, that offered new vocabularies, metaphors, and grammars of suffering.[37] Armed with such interpretive tools, they could begin their journeys forward, stitching together worlds shattered by pain.

# Notes

**INTRODUCTION**

Epigraphs: Woolf [1926] 2002; Wittgenstein [1953] 1973, 89.

1. All names used in this book are pseudonyms.

2. In Chinese medicine, a swollen tongue is indicative of dampness, which generally points to the spleen and may be associated with loose stools, worry, fatigue, or dizziness. "Stuck," in this context, may refer to stagnation, a condition that can affect the $qi$, or blood, and produce pain. I thank Sonya Pritzker for helping me to interpret this assessment.

3. See, e.g., Good 1992, Leder 1990, and Scarry 1985.

4. See, e.g., Desjarlais 1992, Greenhalgh 2001, Jean Jackson 2000, and Throop 2010.

5. For a noteworthy exception, see Crawley-Matoka and True 2012.

6. Rouse 2009, 140. Anthropologists have demonstrated that children's special status and vulnerability is critically shaped by cultural conditions and material constraints. See Scheper-Hughes 1993 and Rosen 2007.

7. Schlegel and Herbert 1991. Anthropologists (e.g., Mead [1928] 2001) have emphasized that Western understandings of adolescence as a transitional, liminal phase of development marked by stress and anguish are culturally and historically contingent. For the purposes of this book, I understand the category to include youth aged eleven to eighteen.

8. Cultural models are schemas that serve as interpretive resources for making sense of the world. In their classic formulation, Quinn and Holland (1987, 4) define cultural models as "presupposed, taken-for-granted models of the world that are widely shared (although not necessarily to the exclusion of other, alternative models) and that play an enormous role in their understanding of that world and their behavior in it." Defining "culture" itself is a trickier business. Contemporary anthropologists no longer think of culture in terms of

discrete and timeless wholes, nor as something that necessarily characterizes a specific group of people in a specific regional setting. Moreover, an important body of work in cognitive anthropology (see, e.g., Garro 2005) about variation within (as well as between) putative cultural groups suggests that we ought to be wary of understanding culture purely in terms of what is shared. In medicine, culture has been construed as a problematic concept because it is often reduced to "ethnicity, nationality, and language" and may be seen to offer an alibi for apparently irrational behavior when other explanations (e.g., inadequate access to resources) are just as plausible (see Kleinman and Benson 2006). My own view of culture emphasizes that culture is a dynamic process rather than a static entity, one that revolves around establishing a more or less shared set of meanings. For a general overview of the critique of the culture concept that is particularly geared toward medical anthropology students, see Lock and Nguyen 2010, 6–9.

9. Farquhar 1996.

10. See, e.g., Byron Good's (1994) problematization of the concept of belief in medical anthropology. According to Good, medical anthropology's romance with notions such as "lay health beliefs" helps to reify an ontological distinction between medical knowledge, which is presumed to reflect the natural world accurately, and lay beliefs, which are presumed to be in some way false or misguided.

11. See, e.g., Evans-Pritchard [1937] 1976, Malinowski 1948, and Rivers 1924.

12. Evans-Pritchard [1937] 1976.

13. *Biomedicine* refers to a particular form of medicine rooted in the Western medical tradition, which emphasizes the scientific, material, and professional grounding of medical knowledge. I use the label *biomedicine* to highlight the cultural and historical plurality of medical systems the world over.

14. For a more thorough overview of these issues, see Good et al. 2010 and Lock and Nguyen 2010, which offer, respectively, an excellent intellectual genealogy of medical anthropology and a survey of the contemporary landscape of the anthropology of biomedicine.

15. Kleinman 1980, 24.

16. See Mattingly 2011.

17. Good 1992, 5.

18. The schematic framework for biomedical explanations that I offer in this section draws on my fieldwork, observations, and personal experiences in U.S. biomedical settings. Although I think that some of these dimensions may be applicable to other settings as well, I do not mean to suggest that biomedicine is the same everywhere. On the cultural formation of biomedicine in the global South, see Wendland 2010 and Livingston 2012.

19. Montgomery 2006.

20. A notable exception is psychosomatic medicine. See Greco 1993.

21. Hamdy 2008.

22. Dumit 2000; Murphy 2006.

23. Peräkylä 1998, 305.

24. Maynard and Frankel 2006, 273.

25. On contestations over medical truth and falsity in an Ayurvedic context, see Langford 1999.

26. Gilbert and Mulkay 1984; Latour 1987.

27. Salmon 2007.

28. Brendel 2003, 569.

29. See Good and Good 1981 for a foundational account.

30. See, e.g. Hunt 1998.

31. Bell and Salmon 2009.

32. Rouse 2009.

33. Farquhar 1996.

34. Throop 2012.

35. See Duranti 1997, 214–44, for a useful anthropologically oriented overview.

36. Keller 2002, 120.

37. My application of Keller's work to clinical medicine should not be taken to mean that Keller's view of scientific explanation only fits the "softer" sciences, however. Within molecular biology, Keller argues, models are representational but are not subjected to truth claims; their value is measured by standards of practical use. She explains, "The notion that a model which is admittedly a fiction can, despite its fictionality, nonetheless capture the features 'of greatest importance' and hence can serve a useful explanatory function has a long and esteemed tradition in these sciences" (Keller 2002, 97).

38. Ibid., 4.

39. On the contingent nature of adjudicating the reality of sensory phenomena, see Austin and Warnock [1962] 1964, 62–77.

40. Good 1994.

41. Foucault [1973] 1994.

42. Most philosophical conceptualizations of dualism do not actually preclude mental and physical causes from interacting with each other. For an introductory philosophical account of the mind/body problem at it applies to mental illness, see Graham 2010, 72–98.

43. Kirmayer 1988.

44. Timmermans and Buchbinder 2013.

45. Although much social theory derides the harmful effects of biomedical uncertainty, my earlier work, as well as that of Whitmarsh et al. 2007, demonstrates that uncertainty may be valuable and generative with respect to specific clinical problems.

46. Trnka 2007.

47. Emily Martin's discussion of the ontology of manic depression is instructive here: "Will I be claiming that manic depression is not 'real'? Not at all. I will claim that the reality of manic depression lies in more than whatever biological traits may accompany it. The 'reality' of manic depression lies in the cultural contexts that give particular meaning to its oscillations and multiplicities" (Martin 2007, 29).

48. Tates and Meeuwesen 2001.

49. Gremillion 2003; Lester 2011; Meyers 2013.

50. See, e.g., Diller 1980, Fabrega and Tyma 1976a, Landar 1967, Pugh 1991, and Throop 2010.

51. Sargent 1984; Throop 2010. See also Zborowski (1952, 1959), who documented variation in the cultural norms guiding the expression of pain in four American ethnic groups.

52. Scarry 1985.

53. Although Scarry's argument is the most widely cited in pain scholarship, similar arguments have been advanced by a number of humanities scholars. David Morris (1991) has suggested, for example, that the natural language of chronic pain is silence.

54. Scarry 1985, 4. See also Good 1992.

55. Asad 2003; Das 1997; Livingston 2012.

56. In developing this claim, Das (1997) employs a thought experiment borrowed from Wittgenstein 1958 in which the reader is asked to imagine whether one person can feel pain in another person's body. For Das, one potential interpretation of this exercise is the possibility that the experience of pain compels the sufferer to seek another to share in its burden. As she puts it, the experience of pain "cries out for this response of the possibility that my pain could reside in your body and that the philosophical grammar of pain is an answer to that call" (Das 1997, 70).

57. Das 1997, 70; see also Das 1998.

58. J. L. Austin ([1962] 1975) classically defined the marriage vow in a wedding ceremony as an "illocutionary" act because the action is accomplished through uttering the words. For applications of the concept of performativity to therapeutic contexts, see Martin 2007, 131, and Carr 2009, 321.

59. Other possibilities include religious frameworks (cf. Asad 2000).

60. Baszanger 1998; Jean Jackson 2000.

61. Rouse 2009.

62. The French neurologist Jean-Martin Charcot introduced a psychological model of hysteria in the late nineteenth century that was later adapted by Freud. In this model, which has been substantially debated and critiqued in the psychoanalytic and feminist literature, a constellation of symptoms, which includes pain and dissociative episodes, is caused by the unconscious mind protecting itself against psychic stress. For an elaboration of this model, see Freud 1989 and Mitchell 2000. For a compelling contemporary response, see Wilson 2004.

63. Nicaraguan women commonly use the term *dolor de cerebro* to refer to pain understood to be caused by persistent worries about the effects of outmigration on the health and well-being of family members remaining behind (Yarris 2009; see also Darghouth et al. 2006).

64. Kirmayer and Young 1998; Kleinman 1986.

65. Lévinas 1988; see also Throop 2010.

66. Beecher 1946.

67. Johansen 2002; Morris 1991; Rey 1995.

68. I thank Harris Solomon for pointing this out to me.

69. Baszanger 1998 provides a helpful overview of Bonica's early work. An extensive anthropological and sociological literature has likewise charted the emergence of specialized pain clinics in the United States (Bates 1996; Corbett

1986; Csordas and Clark 1992; Fagerhaugh and Strauss 1977; Jean Jackson 2000; Kotarba 1983) and Europe (Bendelow and Williams 1996).

70. Wollf and Langley 1968; Zborowski 1952, 1969; Zola 1966.

71. Engel 1977.

72. Some have argued that Engel's conceptualization was too vague and did not actually specify what such a model would look like (e.g., McLaren 1998), while others have suggested that he downplayed the role of power disparities and structural factors in illness processes (e.g., Armstrong 1987). Practically speaking, the biopsychosocial label implies that while psychological factors are recognized to play an important role in pain course and management, they are not (necessarily) assigned a causal role.

73. European Federation of IASP Chapters 2001; Loeser 1991.

74. Institute of Medicine 2011.

75. *Functioning* is a psychological term that refers to one's ability to complete the routine tasks of everyday life. The emphasis on functioning in contemporary biomedical regimes reflects the market logics that aim to restore the sick, as quickly as possible, to their role as productive members of society.

76. Bendelow and Williams 1996.

77. Csordas and Clark 1992.

78. For specific use of this language, see Bates 1996, 143, and Bendelow and Williams 1996, 1130.

79. Corbett 1986; Jean Jackson 1992, 2000.

80. Bates 1996.

81. Institute of Medicine 2011. This report was mandated by an obscure passage in the 2010 Patient Protection and Affordable Care Act. From an anthropological perspective, the report was particularly interesting in light of its call for a change in the "culture" of U.S. pain medicine. Whether such recommendations will receive any traction may still remain to be seen, though Wailoo 2014 is skeptical, given the bleak national economic situation at the time of its release.

82. Wailoo 2014.

83. In the late 1990s and early 2000s, concerns about the abuse of prescription painkillers focused primarily on poor and rural communities. For example, the drug OxyContin was originally dubbed "hillbilly heroin," or "poor man's heroin" because of its popularity in Appalachia. However, it was not long before stories of addicted celebrities and politicians began to roll in, revealing its upwardly mobile, democratizing effects.

84. This is in contrast to other financial schemes for reimbursing physicians, such as capitation, a system in which a fixed amount is paid per patient for a specific unit of time.

85. Stanford et al. 2008; Tsao et al. 2007. These co-morbidities are not unique to pediatric populations, however.

86. Olfson et al. 2014.

87. *Trigger point injections* entail the injection of a small amount of anesthetic into a nerve bundle, usually in the neck, back, or shoulders, but occasionally elsewhere on the body. The anesthetic then numbs the area and loosens the nerve bundles, which can help to relieve myofascial (i.e., muscle tissue) pain.

88. I have struggled considerably over the naming conventions I adopt here. When the clinical team met as a group, the clinicians always called one another by their first names only, including when referring to Dr. Novak or Dr. Petrosian. However, the families typically (with some exceptions) referred to Dr. Novak, Dr. Petrosian, and Dr. Sterling, the psychiatrist, by their professional titles and to others on the team by their first names only. To preserve the hierarchical distinction employed by the families, and to maintain consistency in voice, I refer to the physicians by their professional titles and to the other team members by their first and last names.

89. *Concierge* medicine refers to a trend in U.S. primary care over the past decade in which a patient pays an annual fee in exchange for a higher level of service. In some ways, this is an apt comparison because patients were often faced with out-of-pocket expenses when seeking treatment in the West Clinic. However, these were paid as direct fees for services rendered, rather than through a retainer. In addition, patients whose parents opted against therapies that were not reimbursable could nevertheless remain clinic patients, which would not be true in a luxury clinic, in which all patients are expected to pay an upfront fee. See Brennan 2002 for a discussion of luxury primary care.

90. An HMO (health maintenance organization) is a type of insurance structure in U.S. healthcare in which a single organization manages healthcare for a group of patients who pay a set charge to see physicians belonging to a preestablished network.

91. Greco 2012 argues that the label "medically unexplained symptoms" (MUS) has become fashionable as a way of maintaining neutrality with respect to causal mechanisms and avoiding giving the impression that symptoms are somehow "in the mind." However, Greco points out that this position tends to reify mind-body dualism, which many social scientists working in this area have otherwise worked to disrupt. She explains: "Ideally, we should be able to articulate how the 'mind'—and all that is subsumed in this elusive concept—participates in the production of every type of symptom, and indeed of biomedical disease (Foss, 2002). But the familiar retort that symptoms are 'all in the mind', and especially its use as a way of dismissing symptoms as insignificant or motivated by secondary gain, haunts contemporary discourse on 'MUS' and charges any reference to the psychological character of symptoms with potentially explosive connotations" (Greco 2012, 2367–68).

92. Garro 1994.

93. Chronic regional pain syndrome (CRPS) is a highly debilitating neuropathic pain condition characterized by severe burning pain, restricted range of motion, swelling, and skin sensitivity. While it usually manifests near the site of an injury, it often spreads beyond the original site of damage.

94. Author's field note, October 25, 2008.

95. After Mark's successful trial with neurostimulation, an invasive treatment in which a surgical device is implanted underneath the skin, Julie became fixated on what she viewed as a moral imperative to inform other chronic pain sufferers about neurostimulation. She also tried to enlist me to inform other clinic families about Mark's successful intervention. I tried to explain that as a researcher, I did not feel comfortable advising families on treatment options. This explanation

masked my own skepticism about whether neurostimulation would prove to be a long-term solution for Mark, which it did not. Julie relented somewhat, but she continued to suggest that I might find a way to raise the issue discreetly.

96. See, e.g., Brodwin 2013, Luhrmann 2000, Mol 2003, Rapp 2000, Rhodes 1991, and Young 1995, among others.

97. Buchbinder 2010.

98. Adolescent and parent interviews were designed to elicit basic background information about illness experience, illness history, and treatment-seeking (Groleau et al. 2006) and explanatory models for the onset, treatment, and management of pain (Kleinman 1980); how pain affected the patient's school and social life, as well as broader family processes; and the respondent's thoughts and feelings about the pain. Interviews lasted between one and two hours and usually took place in families' homes, though in a few cases, I met families at a local Starbucks and interviewed them there. Adolescents and parents were almost always interviewed separately. In one case, I interviewed a father-daughter pair jointly at first and then spoke with them separately. In many cases, I interviewed adolescents in family living and dining rooms. I often wondered just how private these settings were, but I always allowed the adolescents and families to choose the rooms for their interviews. Clinician interviews included questions about personal background and pathways to work in pediatric pain management, understandings and explanations of pain, the characteristics of pain patients and their experiences in treatment, and the clinician's approach to pain treatment.

99. I discuss three of these patients in this book: Michael Harris, Mark Siegel, and Claire Joffe. I have omitted the fourth case from this account because the patient did not engage extensively in the West Clinic and her story was ultimately less helpful for illustrating the major themes of this book.

100. See, e.g., Agar 1996.

101. On the epistemological foundations of cases in social inquiry, see Ragin and Becker 1992.

102. This was particularly the case when I received feedback on my work—the manuscript of this book and the journal articles that preceded it—from anonymous reviewers. I am grateful to them for pushing me to clarify the broader significance of my analysis.

103. Livingston 2012, 181. Livingston's case, an oncology ward in Botswana, offers a microcosm of global health, or cancer, or southern African history.

104. Berlant 2007, 666.

105. Jean Jackson 2011, 370.

**CHAPTER 1**

Epigraph: Aristotle, Poetics, trans. S. H. Butcher (New York: Hill & Wang, 1961), 104.

1. Sontag 1978.

2. For anthropological critiques of this position, see DiGiacomo 1992; Scheper-Hughes and Lock 1986, 1987.

3. For a striking example, see Emily Martin's discussion of some immunologists' assertion that the military and warfare imagery so common in scientific models of the immune system "is not just a metaphor but 'how it is'" (Martin 1994, 96).

4. On the failures of testing to erode diagnostic uncertainty, see Timmermans and Buchbinder 2010.

5. "Off-label" use of pharmaceutical treatments refers to medications that are prescribed for use in a way that differs from their U.S. Food and Drug Administration approval, including use for an unapproved indication, age group, or dosage. This practice is legal for physicians, but pharmaceutical companies are not permitted to market drugs for off-label use. Off-label prescribing is extremely common in the United States. See Radley et al. 2006.

6. A *sympathetic nerve block* is an inpatient procedure that involves the injection of an analgesic around the sympathetic nerves in the neck. The objective is to temporarily "switch off" the sympathetic nervous system in order to reduce or eliminate pain.

7. Currently, the American Heart Association recommends that adults maintain a blood pressure of less than 120/80.

8. *Renal artery stenosis* is a narrowing in the renal arteries that restricts the blood flow to the kidneys, leading to impaired kidney function and high blood pressure.

9. Moxa is an herb used in traditional Chinese medicine that produces analgesia when burned on the skin.

10. Medi-Cal is a California Medicaid program that provides health insurance for children and families that meet certain financial requirements and social criteria.

11. Shim 2010.

12. Lucinda was later billed $1,000 for Crystal's gastroenterology visits, although she had not been informed by the gastroenterology clinic in advance that Crystal's treatment would not be covered.

13. Hillary Traynor was not officially part of the West Clinic team, but her office was located in a neighboring metropolitan region, and she received many referrals from the clinic. She often saw patients who lived too far away to see one of the primary psychologists on the team.

14. Rosenberg 2007, 13.

15. In recent years, relatively new diagnoses such as fibromyalgia, multiple chemical sensitivities, and Gulf War syndrome have been mobilized to encompass constellations of symptoms that do not map clearly onto existing disease referents (Barker 2005; Dumit 2000; Murphy 2006). The label *fibromyalgia* was occasionally used in the West Clinic, but it was leveraged cautiously due to the stigma and controversy that the diagnosis has generated (cf. Greenhalgh 2001; Hadler and Greenhalgh 2004).

16. Dumit 2004.

17. On children's use of metaphors and imaginative practices in medicine, see Clark 2004 and Mattingly 2008a.

18. Despite its tremendous influence, Lakoff and Johnson's (1980) argument has been questioned by a number of anthropologists. Strauss and Quinn (1997,

144), suggest, for example, that Lakoff and Johnson attribute too much causal power to metaphor in determining thought and fail to acknowledge the cultural schemas that guide the selection of specific metaphors and enable them to be shared. For a related critique, see Martin 2000, 572.

19. DiGiacomo 1992; Weiss 1997.

20. Scheper-Hughes and Lock 1986, 1987.

21. Garro 1994; Osherson and Rhodes 1981; Martin 1987; Mattingly 2011.

22. Fernandez 1977, 104.

23. Kirmayer 1992, 1994; Rouse 2004.

24. Kirmayer 1993. The philosopher Elisabeth Camp (2009) observes that metaphor is fundamentally pragmatic in that it entails a gap between conventional meanings of words and their use within a specific context.

25. Rhodes 1984. This flexibility is also a liability, as metaphors can lead to misunderstanding when different people interpret them differently. For example, see the discussions by Mattingly (2011) and Rouse (2004) of the different meanings that clinical staff and family members attribute to the "vegetable" metaphor when used to describe a critically ill child.

26. See, e.g., Brodwin 1992, Darghouth et al. 2006, Fabrega and Tyma 1976b, Jean Jackson 2000, 2003, Pugh 1991, and Throop 2010.

27. Dr. Petrosian used this metaphor with almost all of his patients, even if they used an Internet service provider other than AOL. In such a case, he would simply explain, for rhetorical effect, why he chose not to use AOL.

28. On a less hopeful note, the computer metaphor also proved apt for explaining why some kinds of pain turned out to be wholly untreatable: "Some pains may never go away just like some files in your computer, in your CPU, they're there. You can erase them or whatever, but the FBI can come and still pick them out. That means they're still there. There's a residue of them, right?"

29. On the relationship between cultural schemas and individual meaning, see Strauss and Quinn 1997.

30. Mattingly 2011, 370.

31. Osherson and Rhodes 1981.

32. Martin 1994. Martin argues that flexibility itself is a central metaphor for both body and economy in contemporary American culture.

33. Martin 1994, 72.

34. Ibid., 122. Martin elaborates this ideas further, noting, "If you see everything about your health connected to everything that exists but also accept the possibility of managing and controlling at least some of the factors, the enormity of the 'management' task, of controlling one's body and health, becomes overwhelming. Who will manage all this? Is anyone in control?" (123).

35. I thank an anonymous reviewer for pointing this out to me.

36. Kleinman 1980, 110.

37. Rhodes et al. 1999, 1196.

38. Martin 1994.

39. On the role of meaning in therapeutic efficacy, see Kleinman [1973] 2010.

40. Jean Jackson 2000.

41. Ibid., 152.

42. Lakoff and Johnson 1980, 139.
43. Ibid., 144.
44. Becker 1997, 60.

## CHAPTER 2

Epigraphs: Kleinman 1980, 109; Rosenberg 2007, 32. Field notes were constructed at the end of each day of clinic observation based on notes I recorded during the medical consultations. Text enclosed by quotation marks represents discourse transcribed verbatim. Otherwise, extracts from the field notes paraphrase and summarize the clinical interaction.

1. Because CRPS often begins with a broken bone in the arm or leg, it is typical for CRPS patients to be put in a cast many times before a correct diagnosis is made. When the cast is removed and pain remains, orthopedists tend to assume that the bone has not healed properly, and to cast the child again. Unfortunately, immobilization tends to aggravate CRPS, making symptoms worse rather than better.

2. The other clinicians in the West Clinic did not share this precise language in their explanations of pain, although they did agree with Dr. Novak about the characteristics of the prototypical patient.

3. Aronowitz 1998; Beard 1881; Groen 1947.

4. Sontag 1978 describes the romanticization of tuberculosis during the late nineteenth century as a disease of passion that primarily affected creative, sensitive artistic types.

5. Aronoff 1985; Fordyce 1976; Kotarba 1983.

6. Desjarlais 1999.

7. Estroff 1993, 256.

8. The psychiatric anthropology literature offers numerous relevant examples. See, e.g., Carr 2010, Chua 2012b, Davis 2010, 2012, Desjarlais 1999, Kitanaka 2012, Lester 2009, and Luhrmann 2000.

9. LaFontaine 1985; Mauss 1985.

10. See Carr 2010, Lester 2009, Waldram 2012, and Zigon 2010.

11. Geertz 1983, 62–64; Mauss 1985, 14–15.

12. Kleinman 1980. This is an essential, yet often overlooked, aspect of Kleinman's explanatory models framework. While it has often been noted that asking people for their accounts of illness construes the encoding of illness-related knowledge too narrowly (Young 1981; Kirmayer et al. 2004), Kleinman himself suggested that interviews were insufficient for capturing explanatory models and urged researchers to observe practitioners and record their talk.

13. Kleinman 1980, 109.

14. Ibid., 110.

15. Garro 1994.

16. Salmon 2007.

17. Kirmayer 1994, 184–85.

18. Waldram 2000.

19. Moerman 2000.

20. See, e.g., Baer et al. 2008, Casiday et al. 2008, and Garro 1988.

21. Duranti 2010.

22. James [1907] 2010, 62.

23. Casiday et al. 2008.

24. For ethnographic transcription conventions, see the list at the front of the book.

25. See, e.g., Mayer and Tillisch 2011.

26. Park 2010.

27. For a recent account of the opioid epidemic in the United States, see Aviv 2014. For a more critical view of how public health "epidemics" are defined and framed, and what these readings occlude, see Chua 2012a.

28. Suboxone is a compound drug originally developed to treat opiate dependence consisting of buprenorphine and naloxone. For anthropological treatments of buprenorphine, see Campbell and Lovell 2012, Lovell 2006, and Meyers 2013, 2014.

29. The Controlled Substances Act of 1970 and Narcotic Addiction Treatment Act of 1974 restricted replacement therapy to heavily regulated clinical environments for many years. The Drug Addiction Treatment Act of 2000 opened the door for office-based prescription of replacement therapy, albeit in a heavily regulated environment (Campbell and Lovell 2012). During the course of my research, Dr. Sterling conducted Suboxone trials with several West Clinic patients with intricate pharmaceutical profiles. Although Suboxone offered a glimmer of hope for some of the clinic's most challenging cases, it was not always effective at relieving pain, and sometimes introduced problematic side effects. Moreover, when at one team meeting, Rebecca Hunter, the child and family therapist, asked how you could get kids off of Suboxone, Dr. Sterling responded that you might not be able to, noting that it was definitely more of a long-term commitment.

30. For paradigmatic critiques, see Biehl 2007, Healy 2006, and Petryna et al. 2006. I am especially sympathetic to recent approaches that have tried to move beyond a blame-centered form of critique, such as the contributors to the 2014 special issue of *Culture, Medicine, and Psychiatry* on "*Humanness and Modern Psychotropy*," edited by Michael Oldani, Stefan Ecks, and Soumita Basu. As Carolyn Rouse notes in her commentary in this volume, "The authors move beyond castigating global pharmaceutical markets not because there are not tremendous problems with overprescribing, dependence, and overdosing. Instead, they focus on analytic frames that help us unpack why these marginally efficacious drugs are in such high demand" (Rouse 2014, 280).

31. On the Pfizer scandal, see Saul 2008 and Stempel 2014.

32. A striking case was seventeen-year-old Marissa Turkle, who had twice stopped taking all of her medications, without consulting with her doctor, out of fears of dependence and withdrawal. Marissa recounted:

> I don't know why it didn't occur to me, but I was taking pain meds all the time. And then, like after, probably like two months, whenever I wouldn't have 'em in me, I would like start sweating and like shaking and I would, like, feel like I have to throw up. And I was just, like, totally dizzy, and I'm like, this is so weird. And my friend's brother went to rehab for drinking, and so I asked him, I was like, "What does detoxing feel like?" 'Cause it didn't cross my mind until then. And he was like, "Well what

are you feeling," and I told him all of my symptoms, and he goes, "Yeah, you're detoxing." So as soon as I heard that, I stopped taking everything. Like, I wouldn't take anything else. And I detoxed for eleven days.

33. At an earlier point in the interview, Dr. Novak had discussed how hypnotherapy had been an important component of her research and clinical practice.

34. Keller 2002, 120.

35. Kearney and Brown-Chang 2008.

36. The Harrises ended up transferring Michael's psychiatric care to Dr. Sterling early on because Michael's prior psychiatrist proved unreceptive to the West Clinic's holistic, multidisciplinary approach as well as to the idea of communicating with and working as a team. This resistance underscores how unusual the West Clinic's collaborative approach to care might seem within the broader scope of American health care.

37. Risperidone is an antipsychotic medication approved to treat schizophrenia, bipolar disorder, and autism spectrum disorders in children and adolescents. Because it has also been used off-label in children for anxiety disorders, Risperidone was not an unusual medication choice in this context, and does not necessarily indicate that Dr. Novak suspected that Michael had a more serious form of psychopathology. This does not mean that Dr. Novak's choice of this drug was, at the time, entirely uncontroversial, however (cf. Harris 2008). Her reference to a "teeny teeny dose" suggests a desire to downplay potential dangers and minimize the seriousness of this choice. Neither does this choice preclude suspicions that Michael might suffer from an additional psychiatric condition, as I suggest later in the chapter.

38. Vidal 2009, 21.

39. Jon and Sherri had arranged to hold a spot for Zack in a public school in Sherri's parents' school district, since the public school in the Morgans' neighborhood was "not good," according to Jon. Although Jon griped that the tuition at Zack's school had been raised in the midst of a "horrible recession" and said that part of him would be "thrilled" to have Zack move to a public school, he also wanted Zack to be able to attend the same school that his two older daughters had attended through twelfth grade. Jon resented the fact that he had not received better treatment from a school that his children had attended over a seventeen-year period.

40. See Crawford 1994 and DiGiacomo 1992.

41. This technique reflects Allan Young's observation that in their explanations of sickness, individuals exercise "considerable freedom to dissociate, recombine, invoke, or ignore particular elements from occasion to occasion" (1981, 326).

42. Goffman 1959.

43. Kleinman 1980.

44. The advanced placement program offers college level courses at U.S. and Canadian high schools, enabling high-school students to obtain college credit.

45. Lareau 2003.

46. However, familial resistance to the burdens of self-care did not cut neatly across socioeconomic lines, as we will see in later chapters.

47. Rose 2007.

48. Kirmayer 1994.

49. Ibid., 199.

50. Ibid.

51. Kleinman 1980, 223.

52. Lakoff and Johnson 1980, 139. Like Kirmayer 1994 and Brendel 2003, Lakoff and Johnson advocate a pragmatic approach to meaning and truth vis-à-vis these "new," world-changing metaphors: "Though questions of truth do arise for new metaphors, the more important questions are those of appropriate action. In most cases, what is at issue is not the truth or falsity of a metaphor but the perceptions and inferences that follow from it and the actions that are sanctioned by it" (Lakoff and Johnson 1980, 158).

53. See, e.g., Desjarlais 1999, Estroff 1993, Kleinman 1992, Luhrmann 2000, and Ware 1992.

**CHAPTER 3**

Epigraph: Raymaker cited in Ortega 2009, 438. "Nancy Barnes" is a pseudonym for a psychologist outside the West Clinic who was interviewed for this research.

1. For the classifications existing at the time of this study, see American Psychiatric Association 2000. Currently, Rett syndrome is defined as a separate diagnostic category, while the remaining conditions have been subsumed under the single category of autism spectrum disorders (American Psychiatric Association 2013a).

2. See, e.g., Fein 2012, Rose 2007, Rose and Abi-Rached 2013, and Vidal 2009.

3. One psychologist I interviewed made a distinction between PDD, which is a developmental disorder, and psychological disorders. However, because pervasive developmental disorders are listed in the DSM and use psychological diagnostic criteria, I refer to them here as psychological disorders.

4. As anthropologists have noted, diagnostic criteria in general, and these criteria specifically, encode various cultural assumptions—here, about human development and sociality (Daley 2002; Grinker 2008; Ochs and Solomon 2010; Silverman 2008).

5. These disorders were also commonly called autism spectrum disorders; the terms may be used interchangeably. Here, I use *pervasive developmental disorders* to reflect the language employed in the clinic.

6. See, e.g., Eccleston 1995.

7. None of the clinicians I interviewed from outside the West Clinic reported a connection between chronic pain and PDD when I inquired about psychiatric co-morbidities in their patients.

8. Nader et al. 2004; Tordjman et al. 2009.

9. Lester 2007, 382.

10. See, e.g., Douglas 1986 and Bowker and Starr 2000.

11. For example, in her study of American psychiatry, Tanya Luhrmann (2000) shows how the misapplication of such clinical heuristics by novice psychiatrists can result in diagnostic mistakes.

12. As this example suggests, Dr. Novak seemed to have what Bourdieu (1990) has described as a "feel for the game" with respect to PDD diagnosis. This phenomenological awareness was somewhat more opaque to less experienced clinicians.

13. This list served as a material embodiment of what Arthur Frank has called a "road of trials" (Frank 1995, 118) in his depiction of illness as quest.

14. Julie adopted a similarly brazen strategy at Mark's first visit to the physical therapist Sam Carter. While we were sitting in the waiting room in his office, she had been telling me how upset her best friend was about Mark's pain. The first thing that Julie said to Sam when he led us back to the examination room was, "My best friend is counting on you."

15. Julie indicated that Mark had been diagnosed with ADD and not ADHD (attention deficit/hyperactivity disorder).

16. Julie's comfort in making specific requests for prescriptions fits with Annette Lareau's observation that middle-class U.S. parents "act as though they had a right to pursue their own individual preferences and to actively manage interactions in institutional settings" (Lareau 2003, 6).

17. I am indebted to an anonymous reviewer for pushing me to develop this point.

18. Nichter 1981.

19. For recent examples, see Mendenhall et al. 2010 and the articles in Hinton and Lewis-Fernandez 2010.

20. Mendenhall et al. observe: "Idioms of distress are frequently somatic because the language of the body is often a safer or more compelling language than the social or psychological" (2010, 225).

21. See, among others, Grandin 1995, Grinker 2008, Ochs and Solomon 2010, Prince 2010, and Silverman 2008.

22. Lester 2009, 285.

23. See, e.g., Cohen 1998, Lakoff 2005, and Lloyd 2008, as well as the thought-provoking discussion of studying "unformed" objects in Dahlberg 2013.

24. American Psychiatric Association 2013b.

25. See Baron-Cohen 2002. Here "normal" is used to suggest a statistical average rather than a value judgment.

26. Of course, this is not to say that PDD or autism affect only males; the two patients who came to the West Clinic with a previous diagnosis of it were both female.

27. Singh 2013.

**CHAPTER 4**

Epigraph: Foucault [1973] 2006, 99.

1. Cognitive behavioral therapy (CBT) is a structured, directive psychotherapeutic approach that employs a systematic procedure to change patterns of thoughts, feelings, and behaviors (see Waldram 2008). The use of regular homework assignments, in which patients are instructed to implement the techniques learned in therapy in "real life" scenarios, is a hallmark of CBT. Although CBT was accepted as a dominant psychotherapeutic framework in the West Clinic,

and in the larger pediatric pain community more generally, I did hear some clinicians raise concerns at academic conferences about whether all patients were competent to acquire the necessary skills.

2. Anspach 1988, 358.

3. In "The Aetiology of Hysteria," Freud speculated that the repression of childhood sexual trauma could result in psychoneuroses such as dissociation or somatic conversion disorders. Freud later revised his theory, however, when he came to believe that the testimonies of his hysterical patients regarding childhood sexual experiences were motivated by unfulfilled fantasies, and therefore unreliable (Freud 1989). For contemporary accounts of the biopsychosocial pathways linking childhood trauma and chronic pain, see Meagher 2003; Houdenhove et al. 2009. Hart-Johnson and Green 2012 found that among adult chronic pain patients, 70 percent of the men and 65 percent of the women had experienced physical or sexual abuse.

4. Because this chapter deals with sensitive issues such as trauma, some details have been changed for the sake of confidentiality.

5. See, e.g., Lareau 2003 and Ochs and Kremer-Sadlik 2013. Although siblings were in some cases implicated in familial pathology, clinicians generally had much less access to siblings than they did to parents, and siblings were much less involved in pain management strategies.

6. For anthropological perspectives on the clinical production of family roles, see Stryker 2010, Teman 2010, and Thompson 2005.

7. Harkness et al. 2000; Ochs and Izquierdo 2009.

8. Weisner 2002, 273.

9. Suizzo 2004, 315.

10. The discourse of "skills"—and relatedly, "tools"—was widely employed by both families and clinicians in describing therapeutic work. Initially, I was quite suspicious of this language, which seemed to evince a neoliberal logic by which children would be held responsible for their own treatment outcomes. "Tools" and "skills" hold significant appeal within the political economy of U.S. health care, which has moved increasingly toward standardization and evidence-based medicine (Timmermans and Berg 2003). However, as I began to examine the clinic's therapeutic practices more closely, I came to see that there was a great deal more at stake in adolescents' self-care than the language of tools and skills suggests on the surface. Rather, in teaching patients to perform a discrete set of pain management techniques, clinicians were also socializing patients into new ways of thinking, feeling, and acting in relation to distressing experience.

11. Lareau 2003. See also Beatrice Whiting's (1978) earlier discussion of the American "dependency hang-up," the notion that children should be independent within the limiting behavioral structures established by their parents. Such tensions in parental expectations have provided particularly rich fodder for anthropological accounts of adolescent socialization. For example, Peter Demerath's (2009, 48) ethnography of a midwestern public high school identified a distinctive combination of "affective support, pressure, and 'pushing'" in the parenting styles of one community.

12. Pinto 2012. See also Lester 2008.

13. Because Elavil has been found to make some existing (but benign) heart arrhythmias worse, the physicians often ordered a baseline EKG before prescribing it.

14. At an earlier meeting, Craig had described a patient who was extremely tense in her throat, instead of her neck, which he had found odd. He suspected some history of abuse or trauma in her past, although the patient had not mentioned it.

15. Lester 2009.

16. Dr. Novak's reference to a "behavioral plan" employs the language of cognitive behavioral therapy. The concept refers to a clinical approach in which family practices are intervened upon through written guidelines that are specific to a particular family context.

17. Mattingly 2010, 57.

18. I thank Jocelyn Chua for pushing me to develop this point.

19. In this situation, it is quite likely that Claire simply felt more comfortable divulging the details of this interaction to Tess than to her parents. This surrogate-parenting role mirrors that which Helen Gremillion (2003) identified in her study of an inpatient eating disorders treatment facility for adolescent girls, in which the treatment team modeled corrective parenting for patients' families.

20. One of my original research objectives was to videotape in patients' homes to see how chronic pain punctuated the rhythms of family life. As it turned out, of the four focal families that I recruited for in-depth, longitudinal study, only the Siegel family and the family that I do not discuss in this book were willing to let me do this; both the Joffe family and the Harris family declined. This contributed to a shift in my research focus. In Claire's case, my exclusion from videotaping in the intimate domestic sphere was later mirrored by Tess Bergman and Charlotte LeFevre's refusal to let me videotape their sessions, suggesting that videotaping was not in Claire's best interest. Tess did permit me to observe a yoga class, however, and Charlotte spoke with me at length about her work with Claire, although I did not observe. While I found these exclusions frustrating, I ultimately came to see them as of a piece with my underlying interest in tracking vulnerability, intimacy, and relations of care.

21. Cohen 1998.

22. Pinto 2011, 380.

23. See, e.g., Heritage and Lindstrom 1998, Fordyce 2014, Mattingly 2008b, and White 2002.

24. MacDonald and Murray 2007, 59.

25. Amy Borovoy explored the importation of this concept into Japanese popular psychology in her ethnography of a Japanese substance abuse support group. Writing about women faced with a substance-abusing family member, she instructively asks, "When does the nurturing behavior that is ordinarily expected of a good wife and mother become part of a destructive pattern? When does it become exploitative?" (Borovoy 2005, 3).

26. Lester 2011, 485.

27. These comments highlight the gendered dimensions of clinical discourses of parent-child enmeshment. Most clinicians I interviewed suggested that it was *mothers* who typically evidenced enmeshment or co-dependency. Claire's case

was unusual in that clinical suspicions focused on Ricky. This may help to explain why Ricky's overprotective behavior was so troubling to the pain team. Not only was it deemed "inappropriate" parental behavior, but it was all the more inappropriate for a father.

28. In her arresting ethnography of heroin addiction in New Mexico's Española Valley, Angela Garcia (2010) argues that biomedical critiques of intergenerational heroin use overlook the familial love that lies at the foundation of this seemingly disturbing practice. Rather than focus on how parents and children collude in each other's injurious behavior, Garcia suggests that we shift our gaze to the forms of care made possible by intense human suffering.

29. Bateson [1956] 1972. For recent applications of double-bind theory in anthropology, see Cattelino 2010 and Redfield 2012.

30. This represents another version of the American dependency hang-up identified by Whiting 1978. Whiting focused on the mixed messages imposed on children—"seek attention from others but be independent and autonomous" (Weisner 2002, 272)—but contemporary American parents appear to face a similar predicament.

31. The implication of this crude joke was that patients needed to be separated from both their parents (the suffix -*ectomy* meaning surgical removal).

32. See, e.g., Lareau 2003.

### CHAPTER 5

Epigraph: Beard 1881, 193.

1. Hall 1904.

2. Harrington 2008. Beard employed the term *neurasthenia*, introduced via Italian and French from Greek roots to mean "lack of nerve strength," in a metaphorical rather than a physiological sense. This is in contrast to the concept of nervous breakdown, used by Albert Adams in 1901 to mean a collapse caused by literal damage to the nerves by outside pressures (Barke et al. 2000).

3. Beard 1869, 217. As this description suggests, rather than being seen as a sign of weakness, neurasthenia was imbued with a positive moral valence due to its association with civility, sensitivity, and refinement. Neurasthenia thus became a mark of social distinction enjoyed by some of the era's most prominent cultural, intellectual, and political figures, including Edith Wharton, William James, and Theodore Roosevelt (Lutz 1991).

4. However, the decline of the concept of neurasthenia in the West coincided with its rise in Asia, and the term has continued to flourish in modern China (cf. Kleinman 1986).

5. The original archetypal Type A personality was a male with high levels of occupational stress that predisposed him to heart attack. In the mid-1950s, two American cardiologists, Meyer Friedman and Ray Rosenman, having observed that people respond differently to the same events, became interested in the stress-related patterns of behavior in their cardiac patients. They first used the term "Type A" with respect to a specific behavioral pattern typified by a competitive spirit and drive to achieve, a persistent desire for recognition and advancement, involvement in activities subjected to time restrictions, a propensity to increase

the speed of execution of physical and mental functions, and extraordinary mental and physical alertness (Riska 2000).

6. Salmon 2007.

7. Young 1980, 133, notes that while the 1959 *Merriam-Webster's Collegiate Dictionary* defined stress as "the action of external forces," this entry was amended sixteen years later to include "a physical, chemical or emotional state that causes bodily or mental tension."

8. Demerath 2009, 29.

9. Davidson 2011; Demerath 2009; Khan 2011; Levine 2008.

10. See, e.g., Robert LeVine 2011 and Schlegel and Herbert 1991.

11. On the ways in which embodied forms of stress may be symptomatic of larger social and economic shifts, see, e.g., Allison 2013, Chua 2011, Han 2011, and Livingston 2009.

12. Anthropologists have been particularly concerned with the ways in which pain may express resistance or ruptures in the social order. However, Robert Desjarlais (1992), among others, has warned, that in advancing a semiotics of bodily distress, we may eclipse the body itself as a site of disorder.

13. See Bruner 1986, Mattingly and Garro 1998, and Ochs and Capps 1996 for some useful starting points.

14. For example, Jean Jackson (2000) compares the communalizing experience of inpatient pain treatment to a religious initiation rite, suggesting that both provide opportunities for radical transformation and personal growth. She thus argues that pain treatment entails a process of "converting" to clinical ideologies. Similarly, Jarrett Zigon (2010) describes how participants in a Russian drug rehabilitation program engage in a process of "stepping over oneself" (*sebya pridetsya perestupat*) to arrive at a new way of living.

15. From a functionalist perspective, health is vital to the social and economic order because the inability to fulfill certain social responsibilities, such as those to one's job or family, disrupts the smooth functioning of society. Illness, in turn, is a form of "sanctioned deviance" because the sick can no longer fulfill the obligation to be productive members of society. Talcott Parsons (1951) suggested that sick people take on a new set of duties in lieu of their normal social roles. The "sick role" thus entails two major rights and two major responsibilities: (1) exemption from normal social roles and responsibilities; (2) exemption from responsibility for being ill; (3) the desire to want to recover; and (4) the obligation to seek professional help to get well, and a willingness to follow the advice of such professionals. That the sick would depend on these exemptions in order to get well ensured that they would fulfill their reciprocal obligations to society. The four dimensions of the sick role thus constituted a self-reinforcing mechanism of social control. Social scientists have criticized the sick role concept for numerous reasons (cf. Burnham 2012), including its limited utility for theorizing chronic illness, in which case "the sick role's spatial and temporal containment of illness becomes untenable" (Varul 2010, 79). Nevertheless, the concept remains useful for highlighting the social contract that exists between a sick person and society.

16. Reflex sympathetic dystrophy (RSD) is an earlier name for the syndrome that later became known as complex regional pain syndrome (CRPS).

17. Such labels were used to describe Jewish families with some frequency, in keeping with the ethnic stereotype, yet they were not limited to the West Clinic's Jewish families.

18. In her cultural history of depression in Japan, Junko Kitanaka (2012) describes the scientific theory of the "Typus Melancholicus," which proposed that those who are serious, diligent, meticulous, and responsible are prone to *overwork,* a local idiom of distress believed to lead to fatigue and depression. Without discounting the local impact of the global biologization of psychiatry, Kitanaka suggests that neurochemical understandings of depression do not resonate with many Japanese people's understandings of mood and affect. Instead, Japanese psychiatrists in the 1960s and 1970s traced the growing epidemic of depression to the introduction of a modern, industrial capitalist work ethic, the growing alienation of the nuclear family, and the proliferation of a work-obsessed melancholic personality. In the twenty-first century, the explanatory discourse on depression mutated once more to link the Typus Melancholicus to societal changes associated with globalization. This time, Kitanaka notes, the discourse became more overtly politicized when workers and lawyers lobbied to hold corporations and the government responsible for the psychiatric breakdowns of hardworking, committed employees.

19. Scheper-Hughes and Lock 1986.

20. This position draws on Margaret Lock's (1986) work on school refusal syndrome in Japan, a phenomenon whose primary signs and symptoms mirrored those facing West Clinic patients: diffuse complaints, like stomachaches, and tests that turn up negative; bullying and social difficulties; and, ultimately, an adolescent's refusal to attend school. Lock argues that individual psychology and family systems alone cannot account for this pattern of behavior; instead, through school refusal, children subtly challenge broader societal pressures and modes of social control. Amy Borovoy, who has written about a similar phenomenon in Japan, suggests that *hikikomori* (literally, "hidden youth," adolescents who shut themselves away in their parents' homes) are "healthy outsiders in a society that makes unhealthy social demands" (2008, 553).

21. See, e.g., Csordas 1994 and Scheper-Hughes and Lock 1987.

22. Moreover, as Sherine Hamdy points out, reading the body in terms of resistance is complicated because "the body cannot be easily equated with a form of discourse, especially as there is no agreement on how exactly this bodily 'text' should be decoded" (Hamdy 2008, 564).

23. Dominus 2012.

24. Harris 1989.

25. Martin (2007, 4) shows how American ideas about illness and its causes are closely connected to ideas about the market and economic life.

26. As Chua (2012a, 220) puts it: "The 'social,' in this case, fails to recuperate the complex 'local worlds' (Kleinman 1992) of individual and intersubjective suffering against the reductive tendencies of official discourse. Rather, bureaucratic institutions, expert cultures, media representations, and everyday rumors reify categories of social pathology around suicide while 'casting a veil of misrecognition over the domain as a whole' (Kleinman et al. 1997, p. xxv)."

## CONCLUSION

1. See, e.g., Davis 2010.
2. Livingston 2012, 181.
3. Scarry 1985, 53.
4. Anspach 1988; Fordyce 2014; Lareau 2003; White 2002.
5. Garcia 2010; Biehl 2005; Livingston 2012.
6. This message tracks with Joel Robbins's (2013) suggestion that the anthropology of suffering, come of age, has perhaps transmuted into an "anthropology of the good," in which concerns for "care," "empathy," "well-being," "the gift," and "hope" are foregrounded above and beyond the plight of the suffering subject.
7. Since 2008, there has been a surge of anthropological interest in the topic of care, spanning terrain as diverse as humanitarian aid (Ticktin 2011), dementia and personhood (Taylor 2008), clinical practice (Fitzgerald 2008; Livingston 2012), and the embedding of illness in kinship relations (Garcia 2010; Han 2011). While recent work has emphasized that care is a social practice (cf. Mol 2008; Bellacasa 2011), the social situatedness of care entails affective pulls as well as technical labor. Care is materialized in bodies and objects—pills, gestures, techniques, a certain kind of touch—yet there remains an intangible component that occupies a space between people, practices, and moments.
8. See Lester 2011 for one noteworthy exception.
9. Notably, it was the Siegel family that gave up on the West Clinic and not the other way around.
10. Charlotte purchased a shark's tooth for Michael Harris while on a vacation. Prior to the trip, Charlotte and Michael had established that the ocean in Cancun, Mexico, where Michael vacationed yearly with his family, was a "safe place" where he could go to establish control over his feelings. When Michael recounted how he had retreated to this place after a tense fight with his brother, he assured Charlotte, "I promise you I can feel [the water]." After her trip, Charlotte presented Michael with the shark's tooth and explained that he could associate it with swimming in the sea to help overcome his anxieties.
11. Lévinas 1985.
12. Michael Jackson 2002, 252.
13. Of course, this was not always the case; a good counterexample is Dr. Petrosian's discussion of Mark Siegel's "sticky brain" at Mark's first West Clinic appointment.
14. I am particularly moved by the following admonition offered by Claudia Strauss with respect to pragmatic arguments: "Sometimes this awareness is taken to extremes and it is implied that everything an interviewee says is deliberately fashioned for a strategic end. . . . This approach to discourse analysis overlooks the extent to which people's talk (as well as less spontaneous cultural texts) is shaped by a variety of considerations: not only the momentary conscious ones but also less conscious intuitions about what is interesting, funny, normal, and right" (Strauss and Quinn 1997, 241).
15. My use of "belief" here highlights the unsettled, contingent nature of pain as an epistemological object. However, see Good 1994 for a critique of the use of "belief" in contrast to "knowledge" in medical anthropological scholarship.

16. Austin [1962] 1975, 100. As Duranti (1997, 221) notes, "This distinction sanctions the notion of language as action and captures the fact that the same sequence of words can perform quite different kinds of acts (in each case, having a different force) and also recognizes that there is something constant ('meaning') across different uses of the same utterance."

17. Several studies have examined the language ideologies governing code-switching between languages when talking about health and disease (Black 2013; Pigg 2001). More generally, the work of Charles Briggs, Cheryl Mattingly, and James Wilce has been particularly inspiring for its integration of insights from linguistic and medical anthropology. See Wilce 2009 and Kuipers 1989 for helpful overviews.

18. Woolard and Schieffelin 1994, 55.

19. Carr 2010; Desjarlais 1996.

20. See, e.g., Brada 2013, an otherwise exemplary article that, without citing specific evidence or further supporting this claim, takes it for granted that "biomedicine's epistemological framework privileges a referential function of language" (438). Wilce (2009) relatedly points out that referring is, in itself, social action, insofar as directing a doctor's attention to a particular object of concern has effects in the world (202).

21. Kleinman [1973] 2010; Montgomery 2006. Though see work by Ochs, Gonzales, and Jacoby (1996) for a perspective on the expressive and generative dimensions of physicists' speech, which suggests that the dominance of referentialist language ideology may be somewhat suspect in the natural sciences too.

22. Aronowitz 2008; Jutel 2009; Rosenberg 2007.

23. Hacking 1986.

24. Timmermans and Buchbinder 2010.

25. Fein 2012. Carr and Smith 2014, which examines how motivational interviewing (MI) is sustained through "a poetics of pause," is another noteworthy example of anthropological work that pushes beyond a referential view of language: "Quite aside from whether MI 'works' in the sense of actually healing or helping people—a topic that has been pursued by many other researchers—our analysis identifies how MI works semiotically, to produce in real-time discursive practice its signature therapeutic principles. Put very simply, MI's poetic pauses do things, precisely because they send messages to clients and onlookers alike about what kind of interaction a motivational interview is" (108).

26. Brada 2013; Gordon and Paci 1997.

27. Miller et al. 2009; Moerman 2002.

28. Bensing and Verheul 2010.

29. Sherman and Hickner 2007.

30. See, e.g., Specter 2011, a fascinating *New Yorker* profile of Ted Kaptchuk, director of the Harvard-wide Program in Placebo Studies and the Therapeutic Encounter, who has built an impressive neuroscientific research career investigating the therapeutic mechanisms of placebo.

31. Kirmayer 2006, 599.

32. Butler 1997; Hill 2008.

33. On the subtle wielding of power through clinical discourse, see Ainsworth-Vaughn 1998, Kuipers 1989, Mishler 1984, Waitzkin 1991, and Wilce

1998. On medicine as a somewhat more blunt agent of social control, see Starr 1982.

34. Conrad 2007.

35. Unni Wikan's call to anthropologists to reach "beyond the words" sounds a cautionary note against "anthropology's romance with words, concepts, text, and discourse" (Wikan 1992, 464–65). Her concern here is that anthropologists may attend too closely to words for their meaning, overlooking the fact that words are also ways of producing effects.

36. Wittgenstein [1953] 1973, 1, cited in Dumit 2000, 209.

37. Capps and Ochs 1995; Throop 2010.

# References

Agar, Michael. 1996. *The Professional Stranger: An Informal Introduction to Ethnography*. San Diego: Academic Press.

Ainsworth-Vaughn, Nancy. 1998. *Claiming Power in Doctor-Patient Talk*. New York: Oxford University Press.

Allison, Anne. 2013. *Precarious Japan*. Durham, NC: Duke University Press.

American Psychiatric Association. 2000. *Diagnostic and Statistical Manual of Mental Disorders*. 4th ed., rev. Washington, DC: APA Press.

———. 2013a. *Diagnostic and Statistical Manual of Mental Disorders*. 5th ed. Washington, DC: APA Press.

———. 2013b. *Autism Spectrum Disorder*. DSM-5 fact sheets. www.dsm5.org /Documents/Autism%20Spectrum%20Disorder%20Fact%20Sheet.pdf. Accessed December 14, 2014.

Anspach, Renee. 1988. Notes on the sociology of medical discourse: The language of case presentation. *Journal of Health and Social Behavior* 29, no. 4 (December): 357–75.

Armstrong, David. 1987. Theoretical tensions in biopsychosocial medicine. *Social Science and Medicine* 25, no. 11: 1213–18.

Aronoff, Gerald. 1985. *Evaluation and Treatment of Chronic Pain*. Baltimore: Urban & Schwarzenberg.

Aronowitz, Robert. 1998. *Making Sense of Illness: Science, Society, and Disease*. New York: Cambridge University Press.

———. 2008. Framing disease: An underappreciated mechanism for the social patterning of health. *Social Science and Medicine* 67, no. 1 (July): 1–9.

Asad, Talal. 2000. Agency and pain: An exploration. *Culture and Religion* 1, no. 1: 29–60.

———. 2003. *Formations of the Secular: Christianity, Islam, Modernity*. Stanford, CA: Stanford University Press.

Austin, John L. [1962] 1975. *How to Do Things with Words*. 2nd ed. Edited by J. O. Urmson and Marina Sbisà. Oxford: Clarendon Press.

Austin, John L., and G. J. Warnock. [1962] 1964. *Sense and Sensibilia*. Oxford: Oxford University Press.

Aviv, Rachel. 2014. Prescription for disaster. *New Yorker*. May 5.

Baer, Roberta, Susan Weller, Javier García de Alba García, and Ana Salcedo Rocha. 2008. Cross-cultural perspectives on physician and lay models of the common cold. *Medical Anthropology Quarterly* 22, no. 2 (June): 148–66.

Barke, Megan, Rebecca Fribush, and Peter Stearns. 2000. Nervous breakdown in 20th century American culture. *Journal of Social History* 33. no. 3 (Spring): 565–84.

Baron-Cohen, Simon. 2002. The extreme male brain theory of autism. *Trends in Cognitive Sciences* 6, no. 6 (June): 248–54.

Barker, Kristin. 2005. *The Fibromyalgia Story: Medical Authority and Women's Worlds of Pain*. Philadelphia: Temple University Press.

Baszanger, Isabelle. 1998. *Inventing Pain Medicine: From the Laboratory to the Clinic*. New Brunswick, NJ: Rutgers University Press.

Bates, Maryann. 1996. *Biocultural Dimensions of Chronic Pain: Implications for Treatment of Multiethnic Populations*. Albany: State University of New York Press.

Bateson, Gregory. [1956] 1972. Toward a theory of schizophrenia. In id., *Steps to an Ecology of Mind*. Chicago: University of Chicago Press.

Beard, George. 1869. Neurasthenia, or nervous exhaustion. *Boston Medical and Surgical Journal* 3, no. 13 (April): 217–21.

———. 1881. *American Nervousness: Its Causes and Consequences: A Supplement to Nervous Exhaustion*. New York: Putnam.

Becker, Gay. 1997. *Disrupted Lives: How People Create Meaning in a Chaotic World*. Berkeley: University of California Press.

Beecher, Henry. 1946. Pain in men wounded in battle. *Annals of Surgery* 123, no. 1 (January): 96–105.

Bell, Kirsten, and Amy Salmon. 2009. Pain, physical dependence, and pseudoaddiction: Redefining addiction for "'nice" people? *International Journal of Drug Policy* 20, no. 2 (March): 170–78.

Bellacasa, Maria Puig de la. 2011. Matters of care in technoscience: Assembling neglected things. *Social Studies of Science* 41, no. 1: 85–106.

Bendelow, Gillian, and Simon Williams. 1996. The end of the road? Lay views on a pain-relief clinic. *Social Science and Medicine* 43, no. 7 (October): 1127–36.

Bensing, Jozien, and William Verheul. 2010. The silent healer: The role of communication in placebos. *Patient Education and Counseling* 80, no. 3 (September): 293–99.

Berlant, Lauren. 2007. On the case. *Critical Inquiry* 33, no. 4 (Summer): 663–72.

Biehl, João. 2005. *Vita: Life in a Zone of Social Abandonment*. Berkeley: University of California Press.

———. 2007. Pharmaceuticalization: AIDS treatment and global health politics. *Anthropological Quarterly* 80, no. 4 (Fall): 1083–1126.

Black, Steven. 2013. Stigma and ideological constructions of the foreign: Facing HIV/AIDS in South Africa. *Language in Society* 42, no. 5 (November): 481–502.

Borovoy, Amy. 2005. *The Too-Good Wife: Alcohol, Co-Dependency, and the Politics of Nurturance in Postwar Japan*. Berkeley: University of California Press.

———. 2008. Japan's hidden youth: Mainstreaming the emotionally distressed in Japan. *Culture, Medicine, and Psychiatry* 32, no. 4 (December): 552–76.

Bourdieu, Pierre. 1990. *The Logic of Practice*. Translated by R. Nice. Cambridge: Polity Press.

Bowker, Geoffrey, and Susan Leigh Star. 2000. *Sorting Things Out: Classification and Its Consequences*. Cambridge, MA: MIT Press.

Brada, Betsey Behr. 2013. How to do things to children with words: Language, ritual, and apocalypse in pediatric HIV treatment in Botswana. *American Ethnologist* 40, no. 3 (August): 437–51.

Brendel, David. 2003. Reductionism, eclecticism, and pragmatism in psychiatry: The dialectic of clinical explanations. *Journal of Medicine and Philosophy* 28, no. 5–6 (October–December): 563–80.

Brennan, Troyen. 2002. Luxury primary care: Market innovation or threat to access? *New England Journal of Medicine* 346, no. 15 (April): 1165–68.

Brodwin, Paul. 1992. Symptoms in social performance: The case of Diane Reden. In *Pain as Human Experience: An Anthropological Perspective*, ed. M. J. Good, P. Brodwin, B. Good, and A. Kleinman, 77–99. Berkeley: University of California Press.

———. 2013. *Everyday Ethics: Voices from the Front Line of Community Psychiatry*. Berkeley: University of California Press.

Bruner, Jerome. 1986. *Actual Minds, Possible Worlds*. Cambridge, MA: Harvard University Press.

Buchbinder, Mara. 2010. Giving an account of one's pain in the medical anthropology interview. *Culture, Medicine, and Psychiatry* 34, no. 1 (March): 108–31.

Butler, Judith. 1997. *Excitable Speech: A Politics of the Performative*. New York: Routledge.

Burnham, John. 2012. The death of the sick role. *Social History of Medicine* 25, no. 4 (October): 761–76.

Camp, Elisabeth. 2009. Metaphor. In *The Pragmatics Encyclopedia*, ed. L. Cummings, 264–66. London: Routledge.

Campbell, Nancy, and Anne Lovell. 2012. The history of the development of buprenorphine as an addiction therapeutic. *Annals of the New York Academy of Science* 1248 (February): 39–124.

Capps, Lisa, and Elinor Ochs. 1995. *Constructing Panic: The Discourse of Agoraphobia*. Cambridge, MA: Harvard University Press.

Carr, Summerson. 2009. Anticipating and inhabiting institutional identities. *American Ethnologist* 36, no. 2: 317–36.

———. 2010. *Scripting Addiction: The Politics of Therapeutic Talk and American Sobriety*. Princeton: Princeton University Press.

Carr, Summerson, and Yvonne Smith. 2014 The poetics of therapeutic practice: Motivational interviewing and the powers of pause. *Culture, Medicine, and Psychiatry* 38, no. 1 (March): 83–114.

Casiday, Rachel, A.P.S. Hungin, Charles Cornford, Niek de Wit, and Mwenza Blell. 2008. GPs' explanatory models for irritable bowel syndrome: A mismatch with patient models? *Family Practice* 26, no. 1 (February): 34–39.

Cattelino, Jessica. 2010. The double bind of American Indian need-based sovereignty. *Cultural Anthropology* 25, no. 2 (May): 235–62.

Chua, Jocelyn. 2011. Making time for the children: Self-temporalization and the cultivation of the anti-suicidal subject in South India. *Cultural Anthropology* 26, no. 1 (February): 112–37.

———. 2012a. Tales of decline: Reading social pathology into individual suicide in South India. *Culture, Medicine, and Psychiatry* 36, no. 2 (June): 204–24.

———. 2012b. The register of "complaint": Psychiatric diagnosis and the discourse of grievance in the South Indian mental health encounter. *Medical Anthropology Quarterly* 26, no. 2 (June): 221–40.

Clark, Cindy Dell. 2004. Visual metaphor as method in interviews with children. *Linguistic Anthropology* 14, no. 2: 171–85.

Cohen, Lawrence. 1998. *No Aging in India: Alzheimer's, the Bad Family, and Other Modern Things*. Berkeley: University of California Press.

Conrad, Peter. 2007. *The Medicalization of Society: On the Transformation of Human Conditions into Treatable Disorders*. Baltimore: Johns Hopkins University Press.

Corbett, Kitty. 1986. Adding Insult to Injury: Cultural Dimensions of Frustration in the Management of Chronic Back Pain. PhD diss.

Crawford, Robert. 1994. Individual responsibility and health politics. In *The Sociology of Health and Illness: Critical Perspectives*, ed. P. Conrad and R. Kern, 381–89. New York: St. Martin's Press.

Crawley-Matoka, Megan, and Gala True. 2012. No one wants to be the candy man: Ambivalent medicalization and clinician subjectivity in pain management. *Cultural Anthropology* 27, no. 4 (November): 689–712.

Csordas, Thomas, ed. 1994. *Embodiment and Experience: The Existential Ground of Culture and Self*. Cambridge: Cambridge University Press.

Csordas, Thomas, and Jack Clark. 1992. Ends of the line: Diversity among chronic pain centers. *Social Science and Medicine* 34, no. 4 (February): 383–93.

Dahlberg, Britt. 2013. Studying unformed objects: Reflections on how ethnographies of science and process take shape. *Cultural Anthropology* online, http: //production.culanth.org/fieldsights/349-field-notes-in-july-studying-unformed-objects-reflections-on-how-ethnographies-of-science-and-process-take-shape. Accessed November 14, 2014.

Daley, Tamar. 2002. The need for cross-cultural research on the pervasive developmental disorders. *Transcultural Psychiatry* 39, no. 4 (December): 531–50.

Darghouth, Sarah, Duncan Pedersen, Gilles Bibeau, and Cecile Rousseau. 2006. Painful languages of the body: Experiences of headache among women in two Peruvian communities. *Culture, Medicine, and Psychiatry* 30, no. 3 (September): 271–97.

Das, Veena. 1997. Language and body: Transactions in the construction of pain. In *Social Suffering*, ed. A. Kleinman, V. Das, and M. Lock, 67–91. Berkeley: University of California Press.

———. 1998. Wittgenstein and anthropology. *Annual Review of Anthropology* 27: 171–95.

Davidson, Elsa. 2011. *The Burdens of Aspiration: Schools, Youth, and Success in the Divided Worlds of Silicon Valley*. New York: New York University Press.

Davis, Elizabeth. 2010. The antisocial profile: Deception and intimacy in Greek psychiatry. *Cultural Anthropology* 25, no. 1 (February): 1301–64.

———. 2012. *Bad Souls: Madness and Responsibility in Modern Greece*. Durham, NC: Duke University Press.

Demerath, Peter. 2009. *Producing Success: The Culture of Personal Advancement in an American High School*. Chicago: University of Chicago Press.

Desjarlais, Robert. 1992. *Body and Emotion: The Aesthetics of Illness and Healing in the Nepal Himalayas*. Philadelphia: University of Pennsylvania Press.

———. 1996. The office of reason: On the politics of language and agency in a shelter for the "homeless mentally ill." *American Ethnologist* 23, no. 4 (November): 880–900.

———. 1999. The makings of personhood in a shelter for people considered homeless. *Ethos* 27, no. 4: 466–89.

DiGiacomo, Susan M. 1992. Metaphor as illness: Postmodern dilemmas in the representation of body, mind, and disorder. *Medical Anthropology* 14, no. 1 (March) 109–37.

Diller, Anthony. 1980. Cross-cultural pain semantics. *Pain* 9, no. 1 (August): 9–26.

Dominus, Susan. 2012. What happened to the girls in Le Roy. *New York Times*, March 7.

Douglas, Mary. 1986. *How Institutions Think*. Syracuse, NY: Syracuse University Press.

Dumit, Joseph. 2000. When explanations rest: "Good-enough" brain science and the new sociomedical disorders. In *Living and Working with the New Medical Technologies*, ed. M. Lock, A. Young, and A. Cambrosio, 209–32. Cambridge: Cambridge University Press.

———. 2004. *Picturing Personhood: Brain Scans and Biomedical Identity*. Princeton: Princeton University Press.

Duranti, Alessandro. 1997. *Linguistic Anthropology*. Cambridge: Cambridge University Press.

———. 2010. Husserl, intersubjectivity and anthropology. *Anthropological Theory* 10, no. 1–2 (March): 16–35.

Eccleston, Chris. 1995. The attentional control of pain: Methodological and theoretical concerns. *Pain* 63, no. 1 (October): 3–10.

Engel, George. 1977. The need for a new medical model: A challenge for biomedicine. *Science* 196, no. 4286 (April): 129–36.

Estroff, Sue. 1993. Identity, disability, and schizophrenia: The problem of chronicity. In *Knowledge, Power, and Practice: The Anthropology of Medicine and Everyday Life*, ed. S. Lindenbaum and M. Lock, 247–86. Berkeley: University of California Press.

European Federation of IASP Chapters. 2001. EFIC's Declaration on Pain: Pain is a major health problem, a disease in its own right. www.efic.org/index .asp?sub=724B97A2EjBu1C. Accessed November 15, 2014.

Evans-Pritchard, E. E. [1937] 1976. *Witchcraft, Oracles, and Magic Among the Azande*. Oxford: Clarendon Press.

Fabrega, Horacio, and Stephen Tyma. 1976a. Culture, language, and the shaping of illness: An illustration based on pain. *Journal of Psychosomatic Research* 20, no. 4: 323–37.

———. 1976b Language and cultural influences in the description of pain. *British Journal of Medical Psychology* 49, no. 4 (December): 349–71.

Fagerhaugh, Shizuko, and Anselm Strauss. 1977. *Politics of Pain Management: Staff-Patient Interactions*. Menlo Park, CA: Addison Wesley.

Farquhar, Judith. 1996. *Knowing Practice: The Clinical Encounter of Chinese Medicine*. Boulder, CO: Westview Press.

Fein, Elizabeth. 2012. Innocent machines: Asperger's syndrome and the neurostructural self. In *Sociological Reflections on the Neurosciences*, ed. M. Pickersgill and I. Van Keulen, 27–49. Bingley, U.K.: Emerald Group.

Fernandez, James. 1977. The performance of ritual metaphors. In *The Social Use of Metaphor: Essays on the Anthropology of Rhetoric*, ed. J. D. Sapir and J. C. Crocker, 100–131. Philadelphia: University of Pennsylvania Press.

Fitzgerald, Ruth. 2008. Rural nurse specialists: Clinical practice and the politics of care. *Medical Anthropology* 27, no. 3 (September): 257–82.

Fordyce, Lauren. 2014. When bad mothers lose good babies: Understanding fetal and infant mortality case reviews. *Medical Anthropology* 33, no. 5: 379–94.

Fordyce, William. 1976. *Behavioral Methods for Chronic Pain and Illness*. Saint Louis, MO: C. V. Mosby.

Foss, Laurence. 2002. *The End of Modern Medicine: Biomedical Science under a Microscope*. New York: State University of New York Press.

Foucault, Michel. [1973] 1994. *The Birth of the Clinic: An Archaeology of Medical Perception*. New York: Vintage Books.

———. [1973] 2006. *Psychiatric Power: Lectures at the Collège de France, 1973–1974*. Edited by Jacques LaGrange. Translated by Graham Burchnell. New York: Picador.

Frank, Arthur. 1995. *The Wounded Storyteller: Body, Illness, Ethics*. Chicago: University of Chicago Press.

Freud, Sigmund. 1989. *The Freud Reader*. Edited by Peter Gay. New York: Norton.

Garcia, Angela. 2010. *The Pastoral Clinic: Addiction and Dispossession along the Rio Grande*. Berkeley: University of California Press.

Garro, Linda. 1988. Explaining high blood pressure: Variation in knowledge about illness. *American Ethnologist* 15, no. 1 (February): 98–119.

———. 1994. Narrative representations of chronic illness experience: Cultural models of illness, mind, and body in stories concerning the temperomandibular joint (TMJ). *Social Science and Medicine* 38, no. 6 (March): 775–88.

———. 2005. "Effort after meaning" in everyday life. In *A Companion to Psychological Anthropology: Modernity and Psychocultural Change*, ed. C. Casey and R. Edgerton, 48–71. Malden, MA: Wiley-Blackwell.

Geertz, Clifford. 1983. *Local Knowledge: Further Essays in Interpretive Anthropology*. New York: Basic Books.

Gilbert, Nigel, and Michael Mulkay. 1984. *Opening Pandora's Box: A Sociological Analysis of Scientists' Discourse*. Cambridge: Cambridge University Press.

Goffman, Erving. 1959. *The Presentation of Self in Everyday Life*. Garden City, NY: Doubleday Anchor Books.

Good, Byron. 1992. A body in pain—the making of a world of chronic pain. In *Pain as Human Experience: An Anthropological Perspective*, ed. M. J. Good, P. Brodwin, B. Good, and A. Kleinman, 29–48. Berkeley: University of California Press.

———. 1994. *Medicine, Rationality, and Experience: An Anthropological Perspective*. Cambridge: Cambridge University Press.

Good, Byron, and Mary-Jo DelVecchio Good. 1981 The meaning of symptoms: A cultural hermeneutic model for clinical practice. In *The Relevance of Social Science for Medicine: Culture, Illness, and Healing*, ed. L. Eisenberg and A. Kleinman, 165–96. Boston: D. Reidel.

Good, Byron, Michael Fischer, Sarah Willen, and Mary-Jo DelVecchio Good, eds. 2010. *A Reader in Medical Anthropology: Theoretical Trajectories, Emergent Realities*. Malden, MA: Wiley-Blackwell.

Gordon, Deborah, and Eugenio Paci. 1997. Disclosure practices and cultural narratives: Understanding concealment and silence around cancer in Tuscany, Italy. *Social Science and Medicine* 44, no. 10 (May): 1433–52.

Graham, George. 2010. *The Disordered Mind: An Introduction to Philosophy of Mind and Mental Illness*. New York: Routledge.

Grandin, Temple. 1995. *Thinking in Pictures: and Other Reports on My Life with Autism*. New York: Doubleday.

Greco, Monica. 1993. Psychosomatic subjects and "the duty to be well": Personal agency within medical rationality. *Economy and Society* 22, no. 3: 357–72.

———. 2012. The classification and nomenclature of "medically unexplained symptoms": Conflict, performativity, and critique. *Social Science and Medicine* 75, no. 12 (December): 2362–69.

Greenhalgh, Susan. 2001. *Under the Medical Gaze: Facts and Fictions of Chronic Pain*. Berkeley: University of California Press.

Gremillion, Helen. 2003. *Feeding Anorexia: Gender and Power at a Treatment Center*. Durham, NC: Duke University Press.

Grinker, Roy Richard. 2008. *Unstrange Minds: Remapping the World of Autism*. New York: Basic Books.

Groen, J. 1947. Psychogenesis and psychotherapy of ulcerative colitis. *Psychosomatic Medicine* 9, no. 3 (May-June): 151–74.

Groleau, Danielle, Allan Young, and Laurence Kirmayer. 2006. The McGill Illness Narrative Interview (MINI): An interview schedule to elicit meanings and modes of reasoning related to illness experience. *Transcultural Psychiatry* 43, no. 4 (December): 671–91.

Hacking, Ian. 1986. Making up people. In *Reconstructing Individualism*, ed. T. Heller, S. Morton, and D. E. Wellbery. Stanford, CA: Stanford University Press.

Hadler, N. M., and S. Greenhalgh. 2005. Labeling woefulness: The social construction of fibromyalgia. *Spine* 30, no. 1 (January): 1–4.

Hall, G. Stanley. 1904. *Adolescence: Its Psychology and Its Relations to Physiology, Anthropology, Sociology, Sex, Crime, Religion, and Education.* New York: Appleton.

Hamdy, Sherine. 2008. When the state and your kidneys fail: Political etiologies in an Egyptian dialysis ward. *American Ethnologist* 35, no. 4 (November): 553–69.

Han, Clara. 2011. Symptoms of another life: Time, possibility, and domestic relations in Chile's credit economy. *Cultural Anthropology* 26, no. 1 (February): 7–32.

Harkness, Sarah, Charles Super, and Nathalie van Tijen. 2000. Individualism and the "Western mind" reconsidered: American and Dutch parents' ethnotheories of the child. *New Directions for Child and Adolescent Development* 87 (Spring): 23–39.

Harrington, Anne. 2008. *The Cure Within: A History of Mind-Body Medicine.* New York: Norton.

Harris, Gardiner. 2008. Use of antipsychotics in children is criticized. *New York Times*, November 18.

Harris, Grace. 1989. Mechanisms and morality in patients' views of illness and injury. *Medical Anthropology Quarterly* 3, no. 1 (March): 3–21.

Hart-Johnson, Tamera, and Cameron Green. 2012. The impact of sexual or physical abuse history on pain-related outcomes among blacks and whites with chronic pain: Gender influence. *Pain Medicine* 13, no. 2 (February): 229–42.

Healy, David. 2006. *Let Them Eat Prozac: The Unhealthy Relationship Between the Pharmaceutical Industry and Depression.* New York: New York University Press.

Heritage, John, and Anna Lindstrom. 1998. Motherhood, medicine, and morality: Scenes from a medical encounter. *Research on Language and Social Interaction* 31, no. 3&4: 397–438.

Hill, Jane. 2008. *The Everyday Language of White Racism.* Malden, MA: Wiley-Blackwell.

Hinton, Devon, and Roberto Lewis-Fernandez, eds. 2010. *Trauma and Idioms of Distress.* Special Issue of *Culture, Medicine and Psychiatry* 34, no. 2.

Houdenhove, Boudewijn van, Patrick Luyten, and Ulrich Tiber Egle. 2009. The role of childhood trauma in chronic pain and fatigue. In *Trauma and Physical Health: Understanding the Effects of Extreme Stress and of Psychological Harm*, ed. Victoria Banyard, Valerie Edwards, and Kathleen Kendall-Tackett, 37–64. London: Routledge.

Hunt, Linda. 1998. Moral reasoning and the meaning of cancer: Causal explanations of oncologists and patients in Southern Mexico. *Medical Anthropology Quarterly* 12, no. 3 (September): 298–318.

Institute of Medicine of the National Academies. 2011. *Relieving Pain in America: A Blueprint for Transforming Prevention, Care, Education, and Research.* Washington, DC: National Academies Press.

Jackson, Jean. 1992. "After a while no one believes you": Real and unreal pain. In *Pain as Human Experience: An Anthropological Perspective*, ed. M. J. Good, P. Brodwin, B. Good, and A. Kleinman, 138–68. Berkeley: University of California Press.

———. 2000. *"Camp Pain": Talking with Chronic Pain Patients*. Philadelphia: University of Pennsylvania Press.

———. 2003. Translating the pain experience. In *Translation and Ethnography: The Anthropological Challenge of Intercultural Understanding*, ed. T. Maranhao and B. Streck, 172–94. Tucson: University of Arizona Press.

———. 2011. Pain and bodies. In *A Companion to the Anthropology of the Body and Embodiment*, ed. F. E. Mascia-Lees, 370–87. Malden, MA: Blackwell.

Jackson, Michael. 2002. *The Politics of Storytelling: Violence, Transgression, and Intersubjectivity*. Copenhagen: Museum Tusculanum Press.

James, William. [1907] 2010. *Pragmatism*. Las Vegas: Lits.

Johansen, R. Elise B. 2002. Pain as a counterpoint to culture: Toward an analysis of pain associated with infibulation among Somali immigrants in Norway. *Medical Anthropology Quarterly* 16, no. 3 (September): 312–40.

Jutel, Annemarie. 2009. Sociology of diagnosis: A preliminary review. *Sociology of Health and Illness* 31, no. 2 (March): 278–99.

Kearney, David, and Janelle Brown-Chang. 2008. Complementary and alternative medicine for IBS in adults: Mind-body interventions. *Nature Reviews: Gastroenterology and Hepatology* 5, no. 11 (November): 624–36.

Keller, Evelyn Fox. 2002. *Making Sense of Life: Explaining Biological Development with Models, Metaphors, and Machines*. Cambridge, MA: Harvard University Press.

Khan, Shamus Rahman. 2011. *Privilege: The Making of An Adolescent Elite at St. Paul's School*. Princeton, NJ: Princeton University Press.

Kirmayer, Laurence. 1988. Mind and body as metaphors: Hidden values in biomedicine. In *Biomedicine Examined*, ed. M. Lock and D. Gordon, 57–94. Dordrecht: Kluwer Academic.

———. 1992. The body's insistence on meaning: Metaphor as presentation and representation in illness experience. *Medical Anthropology Quarterly* 6, no. 4 (December): 323–46.

———. 1993. Healing and the invention of metaphor: The effectiveness of symbols revisited. *Culture, Medicine, and Psychiatry* 17, no. 2 (June): 161–95.

———. 1994. Improvisation and authority in illness meaning. *Culture, Medicine, and Psychiatry* 18, no. 2 (June): 183–214.

———. 2006. Toward a medicine of the imagination. *New Literary History* 37, no. 3 (Summer): 583–601.

Kirmayer, Laurence, Danielle Groleau, Karl Looper, and Melissa Dao. 2004. Explaining medically unexplained symptoms. *Canadian Journal of Psychiatry* 49, no. 10 (October): 663–72.

Kirmayer, Laurence, and Allan Young 1998. Culture and somatization: Clinical, epidemiological, and ethnographic perspectives. *Psychosomatic Medicine* 60, no. 4 (July–August): 420–30.

Kitanaka, Junko. 2012. *Depression in Japan: Psychiatric Cures for a Society in Distress*. Princeton, NJ: Princeton University Press.

Kleinman, Arthur. 1980. *Patients and Healers in the Context of Culture: An Exploration of the Borderland between Anthropology, Medicine, and Psychiatry.* Berkeley: University of California Press.

———. 1986. *Social Origins of Distress and Disease: Depression, Neurasthenia, and Pain in Modern China.* New Haven, CT: Yale University Press.

———. 1992. Pain and resistance: The delegitimation and relegitimation of local worlds. In *Pain as Human Experience: An Anthropological Perspective,* ed. M. J. Good, P. Brodwin, B. Good, and A. Kleinman, 169–97. Berkeley: University of California Press.

———. [1973] 2010. Medicine's symbolic reality: On a central problem in the philosophy of medicine. In *A Reader in Medical Anthropology: Theoretical Trajectories, Emergent Realities,* ed. B. Good, M. Fischer, S. Willen, and M. J. Good, 85–90. Malden, MA: Wiley-Blackwell.

Kleinman, Arthur, and Peter Benson. 2006. Anthropology in the clinic: The problem of cultural competency and how to fix it. *PLoS Medicine* 3, no. 10: e294.

Kleinman, Arthur, Veena Das, and Margaret Lock. 1997. Introduction. In *Social Suffering,* ed. A. Kleinman, V. Das, and M. Lock, ix–xxvii. Berkeley: University of California Press.

Kotarba, Joseph. 1983. *Chronic Pain: Its Social Dimensions.* Beverly Hills, CA: Sage.

Kuipers, Joel. 1989. "Medical discourse" in anthropological context: Views of language and power. *Medical Anthropology Quarterly* 3, no. 2 (June): 99–123.

LaFontaine, J. S. 1985. Person and individual. In *The Category of the Person: Anthropology, Philosophy, History,* ed. M. Carrithers, S. Collins, and S. Lukes, 123–40. Cambridge: Cambridge University Press.

Lakoff, Andrew. 2005. *Pharmaceutical Reason: Knowledge and Value in Global Psychiatry.* Cambridge: Cambridge University Press.

Lakoff, George, and Mark Johnson. 1980. *Metaphors We Live By.* Chicago: University of Chicago Press.

Landar, Herbert. 1967. The language of pain in Navaho culture. In *Studies in Southwestern Ethnolinguistics,* ed. D. H. Hymes and W. E. Bittle, 117–44. Paris: Mouton.

Langford, Jean. 1999. Medical mimesis: healing signs of a cosmopolitan "quack." *American Ethnologist* 26, no. 1 (February): 24–46.

Lareau, Annette. 2003. *Unequal Childhoods: Class, Race, and Family Life.* Berkeley: University of California Press.

Latour, Bruno. 1987. *Science in Action: How to Follow Scientists and Engineers Through Society.* Cambridge, MA: Harvard University Press.

Leder, Drew. 1990. *The Absent Body.* Chicago: University of Chicago Press.

Lester, Rebecca. 2007. Critical therapeutics: Cultural politics and clinical reality in two eating disorder treatment centers. *Medical Anthropology Quarterly* 21, no. 4 (December): 369–87.

———. 2008. Anxious bliss: A case study of dissociation in a Mexican nun. *Transcultural Psychiatry* 45, no. 1 (March): 56–78.

———. 2009. Brokering authenticity: Borderline personality disorder and the ethics of care in an American eating disorder clinic. *Current Anthropology* 50, no. 3 (June): 281–302.

———. 2011. How do I code for black fingernail polish? Finding the missing adolescent in managed mental health care. *Ethos* 39, no. 4 (December): 481–96.

Lévinas, Emmanuel. 1985. *Ethics and Infinity*. Translated by R. Cohen. Pittsburgh: Duquesne University Press.

———. 1988. Useless Suffering. In *The Provocation of Levinas: Rethinking the Other*, ed. R. Bernasconi and D. Wood. Routledge: New York.

Levine, Madeline. 2008. *The Price of Privilege: How Parental Pressure and Material Advantage are Creating a Generation of Disconnected and Unhappy Kids*. New York: Harper Perennial.

LeVine, Robert. 2011. Traditions in transition: Adolescents remaking culture. *Ethos* 39, no. 4 (December): 426–31.

Lévi-Strauss, Claude. 1963. The sorcerer and his magic. In id., *Structural Anthropology*, 167–85. New York: Basic Books.

Livingston, Julie. 2009. Suicide, risk, and investment in the heart of the African miracle. *Cultural Anthropology* 24: 652–80.

———. 2012. *Improvising Medicine: An African Oncology Ward in an Emerging Epidemic*. Durham, NC: Duke University Press.

Lloyd, Stephanie. 2008. Morals, medicine, and change: Morality brokers, social phobias, and French psychiatry. *Culture, Medicine, and Psychiatry* 32, no. 2 (June): 279–97.

Lock, Margaret. 1986. Plea for acceptance: School refusal syndrome in Japan. *Social Science and Medicine* 23, no. 2: 99–112.

Lock, Margaret, and Vinh-Kim Nguyen. 2010. *An Anthropology of Biomedicine*. Malden, MA: Wiley-Blackwell.

Loeser, John. 1991. What is chronic pain? *Theoretical Medicine* 12, no. 2: 213–25.

Lovell, Anne. 2006. Addiction markets: The case of high-dose buprenorphine in France. In *Global Pharmaceuticals: Ethics, Markets, Practices*, ed. A. Petryna, A. Lakoff, and A. Kleinman, 136–70. Durham, NC: Duke University Press.

Luhrmann, T. M. 2000. *Of Two Minds: The Growing Disorder in American Psychiatry*. New York: Knopf.

Lutz, Tom. 1991. *American Nervousness, 1903: An Anecdotal History*. Ithaca, NY: Cornell University Press.

MacDonald, Mary Ellen, and Mary Ann Murray. 2007. The appropriateness of appropriate: Smuggling values into clinical practice. *Canadian Journal of Nursing Research* 39, no. 4 (December): 58–73.

Malinowski, Bronislaw. 1948. *Magic, Science, and Religion and Other Essays*. Garden City, New York: Doubleday Anchor books.

Martin, Emily. 1987. *The Woman in the Body: A Cultural Analysis of Reproduction*. Boston: Beacon Press.

———. 1994. *Flexible Bodies: The Role of Immunity in American Culture from the days of Polio to the Age of AIDS*. Boston: Beacon Press.

———. 2000. Mind-body problems. *American Ethnologist* 27, no. 3 (August): 569–90.

———. 2007. *Bipolar Expeditions: Mania and Depression in American Culture.* Princeton, NJ: Princeton University Press.

Mattingly, Cheryl. 2008a. Pocahontas goes to the clinic: Popular culture as lingua franca. *American Anthropologist* 108, no. 3 (April): 494–501.

———. 2008b. Reading minds and telling tales in a cultural borderland. *Ethos* 36, no.1 (March): 136–54.

———. 2010. *The Paradox of Hope: Journeys through a Clinical Borderland.* Berkeley: University of California Press.

———. 2011. The machine-body as contested metaphor in clinical care. *Genres* 44, no. 3: 363–80.

Mattingly, Cheryl, and Linda Garro, eds. 1998. *Narrative and the Cultural Construction of Illness and Healing.* Berkeley: University of California Press.

Mauss, Marcel. [1938] 1985. A category of the human mind: The notion of the person, the notion of the self. In *The Category of the Person: Anthropology, Philosophy, History,* ed. M. Carrithers, S. Collins, and S. Lukes, 1–25. Cambridge: Cambridge University Press.

Mayer, Emeran, and Kirsten Tillisch. 2011. The brain-gut axis in abdominal pain syndromes. *Annual Review of Medicine* 62: 381–96.

Maynard, Douglas, and Richard Frankel. 2006. On diagnostic rationality: Bad news, good news, and the symptom residue. In *Communication in Medical Care: Interaction Between Primary Care Physicians and Patients,* ed. J. Heritage and D. Maynard, 248–78. Cambridge: Cambridge University Press.

McLaren, Niall. 1998. A critical review of the biopsychosocial model. *Australian and New Zealand Journal of Psychiatry* 32, no. 1 (February): 86–92.

Mead, Margaret. [1928] 2001. *Coming of Age in Samoa: A Psychological Study of Primitive Youth for Western Civilization.* New York: Harper Collins.

Meagher, Mary. 2003. Links between traumatic family violence and chronic pain: Biopsychosocial pathways and treatment implications. In *Health Consequences of Abuse in the Family: A Clinical Guide for Evidence-Based Practice,* ed. Kathleen Kendall-Tackett, 155–78. Washington, DC: American Psychological Association.

Mendenhall, Emily, Rebecca Seligman, Alicia Fernandez, and Elizabeth Jacobs. 2010. Speaking through diabetes: Rethinking the significance of lay discourses on diabetes. *Medical Anthropology Quarterly* 24, no. 2 (June): 220–39.

Meyers, Todd. 2013. *The Clinic and Elsewhere: Addiction, Adolescents and the Afterlife of Therapy.* Seattle: University of Washington Press.

———. 2014. Promise and deceit: Pharmakos, drug replacement therapy, and the perils of experience. *Culture, Medicine, and Psychiatry* 38, no. 2 (June): 182–96.

Miller, Franklin, Luana Colloca, and Ted Kaptchuk. 2009. The placebo effect: Illness and interpersonal healing. *Perspectives in Biology and Medicine* 52, no. 4 (Autumn): 518–39.

Mishler, Elliot. 1984. *The Discourse of Medicine: Dialectics of Medical Interviews.* Norwood, NJ: Ablex.

Mitchell, Juliet. 2000. *Mad Men and Medusas: Reclaiming Hysteria*. New York: Basic Books.

Moerman, Daniel. 2000. Cultural variations in the placebo effect: Ulcers, anxiety, and blood pressure. *Medical Anthropology Quarterly* 14, no. 1 (March): 51–72.

———. 2002. *Meaning, Medicine, and the "Placebo Effect."* Cambridge: Cambridge University Press.

Mol, Annemarie. 2003. *The Body Multiple: Ontology in Medical Practice*. Durham, NC: Duke University Press.

———. 2008. *The Logic of Care: Health and the Problem of Patient Choice*. New York: Routledge.

Montgomery, Kathryn. 2006. *How Doctors Think: Clinical Judgment and the Practice of Medicine*. Oxford: Oxford University Press.

Morris, David. 1991. *The Culture of Pain*. Berkeley: University of California Press.

Murphy, Michelle. 2006. *Sick Building Syndrome and the Problem of Uncertainty: Environmental Politics, Technoscience, and Women Workers*. Durham, NC: Duke University Press.

Nader, Rami, Tim Oberlander, Christine Chambers, and Kenneth Craig. 2004. Expression of pain in children with autism. *Clinical Journal of Pain* 20, no. 2 (March–April): 88–97.

Nichter, Mark. 1981. Idioms of distress: alternatives in the expression of psychosocial distress: A case study from India. *Culture, Medicine, and Psychiatry* 5, no. 4 (December): 379–408.

Ochs, Elinor, and Lisa Capps. 1996. Narrating the self. *Annual Review of Anthropology* 25: 19–43.

Ochs, Elinor, and Carolina Izquierdo. 2009. Responsibility in childhood: Three developmental trajectories. *Ethos* 37, no. 4 (December): 391–413.

Ochs, Elinor, and Tamar Kremer-Sadlik, eds.. 2013. *Fast-Forward Family: Home, Work, and Relationships in Middle-Class America*. Berkeley: University of California Press.

Ochs, Elinor, Patrick Gonzales, and Sally Jacoby. 1996. When I come down I'm in a domain state: Talk, gesture, and graphic representation in the interpretive activity of physicists. In *Interaction and Grammar*, ed. E. Ochs, E. Schegloff, and S. Thompson, 328–69. Cambridge: Cambridge University Press.

Ochs, Elinor, and Olga Solomon. 2010. Autistic sociality. *Ethos* 38, no. 1 (March): 69–21.

Oldani, Michael, Stefan Ecks, and Soumita Basu, eds. 2014 . *Humanness and Modern Psychotropy*. Special Issue of *Culture, Medicine, and Psychiatry* 38, no. 2 (June).

Olfson, Mark, Carlos Blanco, Shuai Wang, Gonzalo Laje, and Christoph Correll. 2014. National trends in the mental health care of children, adolescents, and adults by office-based physicians. *JAMA Psychiatry* 71, no. 1 (January): 81–90.

Ortega, Francisco. 2009. The cerebral subject and the challenge of neurodiversity. *BioSocieties* 4, no. 4 (December): 425–45.

Osherson, S., and Lorna A. Rhodes. 1981. The machine metaphor in medicine. In *Social Contexts of Health, Illness, and Patient Care*, ed. E. Mishler, L. A.

Rhodes, S.T. Hauser, R. Liem, S.D. Osherson, and N.E. Waxler, 218–49. Cambridge: Cambridge University Press.

Park, Melissa. 2010. Beyond calculus: Apple-apple-ike and other embodied pleasures for a child diagnosed with autism in a sensory integration based clinic. *Disability Studies Quarterly* 30, no. 1 (Winter). www.academia.edu/1530836/ Beyond_Calculus_Apple-apple-apple-ike_and_Other_Embodied_Pleasures_ for_a_Child_Diagnosed_with_Autism_in_a_Sensory_Integration_Based_ Clinic. Accessed December 14, 2014.

Parsons, Talcott. 1951. *The Social System*. Glencoe, IL: Free Press.

Peräkylä, Anssi. 1998. Authority and accountability: The delivery of diagnosis in primary health care. *Social Psychology Quarterly* 61, no. 4 (December): 301–20.

Petryna, Adriana, Andrew Lakoff, and Arthur Kleinman, eds. 2006. *Global Pharmaceuticals: Ethics, Markets, Practices*. Durham, NC: Duke University Press.

Pigg, Stacy. 2001. Languages of sex and AIDS in Nepal: Notes on the social production of commensurability. *Cultural Anthropology* 16, no. 4 (November): 481–541.

Pinto, Sarah. 2011. Rational love, relational medicine: Psychiatry and the accumulation of precarious kinship. *Culture, Medicine, and Psychiatry* 35, no. 3 (September): 376–95.

———. 2012 The limits of diagnosis: Sex, law, and psychiatry in a case of contested marriage. *Ethos* 40, no. 2 (June): 119–41.

Prince, Dawn Eddings. 2010. An exceptional path: An ethnographic narrative reflecting on autistic parenthood from evolutionary, cultural, and spiritual perspectives. *Ethos* 38, no. 1 (March): 56–68.

Pugh, Judy. 1991. The semantics of pain in Indian culture and medicine. *Culture, Medicine, and Psychiatry* 15, no. 1 (March): 19–43.

Quinn, Naomi, and Dorothy Holland. 1987. Culture and cognition. In *Cultural Models in Language and Thought*, ed. D. Holland and N. Quinn, 3–42. Cambridge: Cambridge University Press.

Radley, David, Stan Finkelstein, and Randall Stafford. 2006. Off-label prescribing among office-based physicians. *Archives of Internal Medicine* 166, no. 9 (May): 1021–26.

Rapp, Rayna. 2000. *Testing Women, Testing the Fetus: The Social Impact of Amniocentesis in America*. New York: Routledge.

Ragin, Charles, and Howard Becker, eds. 1992. *What Is a Case? Exploring the Foundations of Social Inquiry*. Cambridge: Cambridge University Press.

Redfield, Peter. 2012. The unbearable lightness of ex-pats: Double binds of humanitarian mobility. *Cultural Anthropology* 27, no. 2 (May): 358–82.

Rey, Roselyne. 1995. *The History of Pain*. Translated by L. Wallace, J. Cadden, and S. Cadden. Cambridge, MA: Harvard University Press.

Rhodes, Lorna A. 1984. "This will clear your mind": The use of metaphor for medication in psychiatric settings. *Culture, Medicine, and Psychiatry* 8, no. 1 (March): 49–70.

———. 1991. *Emptying Beds: The Work of an Emergency Psychiatry Unit*. Berkeley: University of California Press.

Rhodes, Lorna A., Carol McPhillips-Tangum, Christine Markham, and Rebecca Klenk. 1999. The power of the visible: The meaning of diagnostic tests in chronic back pain. *Social Science and Medicine* 48, no. 9 (May): 1189–1203.

Riska, Elianne. 2000. The rise and fall of type A man. *Social Science and Medicine* 51, no. 11 (December): 1665–74.

Rivers, William H. 1924. *Medicine, Magic, and Religion*. London: Routledge.

Robbins, Joel. 2013. Beyond the suffering subject: Toward an anthropology of the good. *Journal of the Royal Anthropological Institute* 19, no. 3 (September): 447–62.

Rose, Nikolas. 2007. *The Politics of Life Itself: Biomedicine, Power, and Subjectivity in the Twenty-First Century*. Princeton: Princeton University Press.

Rose, Nikolas, and Joelle Abi-Rached. 2013. *Neuro: The New Brain Sciences and the Management of the Mind*. Princeton: Princeton University Press.

Rosen, David. 2007. Child soldiers, international humanitarian law, and the globalization of childhood. *American Anthropologist* 109, no. 2 (June): 296–306.

Rosenberg, Charles. 2007. *Our Present Complaint: American Medicine, Then and Now*. Baltimore: Johns Hopkins University Press.

Rouse, Carolyn. 2004. "If she's a vegetable, we'll be her garden": Embodiment, transcendence, and citations of competing cultural metaphors in the case of a dying child. *American Ethnologist* 31, no. 4 (November): 514–29.

———. 2009. *Uncertain Suffering: Racial Health Care Disparities and Sickle Cell Disease*. Berkeley: University of California Press.

———. 2014. Cultural scripts: The elusive role of psychotropic drugs in treatment. *Culture, Medicine, and Psychiatry* 38, no. 2 (June): 279–82.

Salmon, Peter. 2007. Conflict, collusion, or collaboration in consultations about medically unexplained symptoms: The need for a curriculum of medical explanation. *Patient Education and Counseling* 67, no. 3 (August): 246–54.

Sargent, Carolyn. 1984. Between death and shame: Dimensions of pain in Bariba culture. *Social Science and Medicine* 19, no. 12: 1299–1304.

Saul, Stephanie. 2008. Experts conclude Pfizer manipulated studies. *New York Times*, October 8.

Scarry, Elaine. 1985. *The Body in Pain: The Making and Unmaking of a World*. Oxford: Oxford University Press.

Scheper-Hughes, Nancy. 1993. *Death Without Weeping: The Violence of Everyday Life in Brazil*. Berkeley: University of California Press.

Scheper-Hughes, Nancy, and Margaret Lock. 1986. Speaking truth to illness: Metaphors, reification, and a pedagogy for patients. *Medical Anthropology Quarterly* 17, no. 5 (November): 137–40.

———. 1987. The mindful body: A prolegomenon to future work in medical anthropology. *Medical Anthropology Quarterly* 1, no. 1 (March): 6–41.

Schlegel, Alice, and Barry Herbert. 1991. *Adolescence: An Anthropological Inquiry*. Free Press.

Sherman, Rachel, and John Hickner. 2007. Academic physicians use placebos in clinical practice and believe in the mind-body connection. *Journal of General Internal Medicine* 23, no. 1 (January): 7–10.

Shim, Janet. 2010. Cultural health capital: A theoretical approach to understanding health care interactions and the dynamics of unequal treatment. *Journal of Health and Social Behavior* 51, no. 1 (March): 1–15.

Silverman, Chloe. 2008. Fieldwork on another planet: Social science perspectives on the autism spectrum. *BioSocieties* 3, no. 3 (September): 325–41.

Singh, Ilina. 2013. Brain talk: Power and negotiation in children's discourse about self, brain and behaviour. *Sociology of Health & Illness* 35, no. 6 (July): 813–27.

Sontag, Susan. 1978. *Illness as Metaphor.* New York: Farrar, Straus, & Giroux.

Specter, Michael. 2011. The power of nothing. *New Yorker*, December 12.

Stanford, Elizabeth, Christine Chambers, Jeremy Biesanz, and Edith Chen. 2008. Frequency, trajectories and predictors of adolescent recurrent pain: A population-based approach. *Pain* 138, no. 1 (August): 11–21.

Starr, Paul. 1982. *The Social Transformation of American Medicine.* New York: Basic Books.

Stempel, Jonathan. 2014. Pfizer to pay $325 million in Neurontin settlement. www.reuters.com/article/2014/06/02/us-pfizer-neurontin-settlement-idUSKBN0E D1IS20140602. Accessed November 15, 2014.

Strauss, Claudia, and Naomi Quinn. 1997. *A Cognitive Theory of Cultural Meaning.* Cambridge: Cambridge University Press.

Stryker, Rachael. 2010. *The Road to Evergreen: Adoption, Attachment Therapy, and the Promise of Family.* Ithaca, NY: Cornell University Press.

Suizzo, Marie-Anne. 2004. Mother-child relationships in France: Balancing autonomy and affiliation in everyday interactions. *Ethos* 32, no. 3 (September): 293–323.

Tates, Kiek, and Ludwien Meeuwesen. 2001. Doctor-parent-child communication: A (re)view of the literature. *Social Science and Medicine* 52, no. 6 (March): 839–51.

Taylor, Janelle. 2008. On recognition, caring, and dementia. *Medical Anthropology Quarterly* 22, no. 4 (December): 313–35.

Teman, Elly. 2010. *Birthing a Mother: The Surrogate Body and the Pregnant Self.* Berkeley: University of California Press.

Thompson, Charis. 2005. *Making Parents: The Ontological Choreography of Reproductive Technologies.* Cambridge, MA: MIT Press.

Throop, C. Jason. 2010. *Suffering and Sentiment: Exploring the Vicissitudes of Pain and Experience in Yap.* Berkeley: University of California Press.

———. 2012 On the varieties of empathic experience: Tactility, mental opacity, and pain in Yap. *Medical Anthropology Quarterly* 26, no. 3 (September): 408–30.

Ticktin, Miriam. 2011 *Casualties of Care: Immigration and the Politics of Humanitarianism in France.* Berkeley: University of California Press.

Timmermans, Stefan, and Marc Berg. 2003. *The Gold Standard: The Challenge of Evidence-Based Medicine and Standardization in Health Care.* Philadelphia: Temple University Press.

Timmermans, Stefan, and Mara Buchbinder. 2010. Patients-in-waiting: Living between sickness and health in the genomics era. *Journal of Health and Social Behavior* 51, no. 4 (December): 408–23.

———. 2013. *Saving Babies? The Consequences of Newborn Genetic Screening*. Chicago: University of Chicago Press.

Tordjman, Sylvie, George Anderson, Michel Botbol, Sylvie Brailly-Tabard, Fernando Perez-Diaz, Rozenn Gaignic, Michele Carlier, Gerard Schmit, Anne-Catherine Rolland, Olivier Bonnot, Severine Trabado, Pierre Roubertoux, and Guillaume Bronsard. 2009. Pain reactivity and plasma beta-endorphin in children and adolescents with autistic disorder. *PLoS One* 4, no. 8 (August): e5289.

Trnka, Susanna. 2007. Languages of labor: Negotiating the "real" and the relational in Indo-Fijian women's expressions of physical pain. *Medical Anthropology Quarterly* 21, no. 4 (December): 388–408.

Tsao, Jennie, Marcia Meldrum, Su Kim, and Lonnie Zeltzer. 2007. Anxiety-sensitivity and health-related quality of life in children with chronic pain. *Journal of Pain* 8, no. 10 (October): 814–23.

Varul, Matthias Zick. 2010. Talcott Parsons, the sick role and chronic illness. *Body & Society* 16, no. 2 (June): 72–94.

Vidal, Fernando. 2009. Brainhood, anthropological figure of modernity. *History of the Human Sciences* 22, no. 1 (February): 5–36.

Wailoo, Keith. 2014. *Pain: A Political History*. Baltimore: Johns Hopkins University.

Waitzkin, Howard. 1991. *The Politics of Medical Encounters*. New Haven, CT: Yale University Press.

Waldram, James. 2000. The efficacy of traditional medicine: Current theoretical and methodological issues. *Medical Anthropology Quarterly* 14, no. 4 (December): 603–25.

———. 2008. The narrative challenge to cognitive behavioral treatment of sexual offenders. *Culture, Medicine, and Psychiatry* 32, no. 3 (September): 421–39.

———. 2012. *Hound Pound Narrative: Sexual Offender Habilitation and the Anthropology of Therapeutic Intervention*. Berkeley: University of California Press.

Ware, Norma. 1992. The delegitimation of illness experience in chronic fatigue syndrome. *Medical Anthropology Quarterly* 6, no. 4 (December): 347–61.

Weisner, Thomas. 2002. The American dependency conflict: Continuities and discontinuities in behavior and values of countercultural parents and their children. *Ethos* 29, no. 3 (September): 271–95.

Weiss, Meira. 1997. Signifying the pandemics: Metaphors of AIDS, cancer, and heart disease. *Medical Anthropology Quarterly* 11, no. 4 (December): 456–76.

Wendland, Claire. 2010. *A Heart for the Work: Journeys through an African Medical School*. Chicago: University of Chicago Press.

White, Susan. 2002. Accomplishing "the case" in paediatrics and child health: Medicine and morality in interprofessional talk. *Sociology of Health & Illness* 24, no. 6 (November): 409–35.

Whiting, Beatrice. 1978. The dependency hang-up and experiments in alternative life styles. In *Major Social Issues: A Multidisciplinary View*, ed. Milton J. Yinger and Stephan J. Cutler, 217–26. New York: Free Press.

Whitmarsh, Ian, Arlene Davis, Debra Skinner, and Donald Bailey Jr. 2007. A place for genetic uncertainty: Parents valuing an unknown in the meaning of disease. *Social Science and Medicine* 65, no. 6 (September): 1082–93.

Wilce, James. 1998. *Eloquence in Trouble: The Poetics and Politics of Complaint in Rural Bangladesh*. New York: Oxford University Press.

———. 2009. Medical discourse. *Annual Review of Anthropology* 38: 199–215.

Wilson, Elizabeth A. 2004. *Psychosomatic: Feminism and the Neurological Body*. Durham, NC: Duke University Press.

Wikan, Unni. 1992. Beyond the words: The power of resonance. *American Ethnologist* 19, no. 3 (August): 460–82.

Wittgenstein, Ludwig. 1958. *The Blue and Brown Books*. London: Basil Blackwell.

———. [1953] 1973. *Philosophical Investigations*. Translated by G. E. M. Anscombe. 3rd ed. Englewood Cliffs, NJ: Prentice Hall.

Wolff, B. Berthold, and Sarah Langley. 1968. Cultural factors and the response to pain. *American Anthropologist* 70, no. 3 (June): 494–501.

Woolard, Kathryn, and Bambi Schieffelin. 1994. Language ideology. *Annual Review of Anthropology* 23: 55–82.

Woolf, Virginia. [1926] 2002. *On Being Ill*. New York: Paris Press.

Yarris, Kristin Elizabeth. 2009. The pain of "thinking too much": *Dolor de cerebro* and the embodiment of social hardship among Nicaraguan women. *Ethos* 39, no. 2 (June): 226–48.

Young, Allan. 1980. The discourse of stress and the reproduction of conventional knowledge. *Social Science and Medicine* 14B, no. 3 (August): 133–46.

———. 1981. When rational men fall sick: An inquiry into some assumptions made by medical anthropologists. *Culture, Medicine, and Psychiatry* 5, no. 4 (December): 317–35.

———. 1995. *The Harmony of Illusions: Inventing Post-Traumatic Stress Disorder*. Princeton: Princeton University Press.

Zborowski, Mark. 1952. Cultural components in response to pain. *Journal of Social Issues* 8, no. 4 (Fall): 16–30.

———. 1969. *People in Pain*. San Francisco: Jossey-Bass.

Zigon, Jarrett. 2010. *"HIV is God's Blessing": Rehabilitating Morality in Neoliberal Russia*. Berkeley: University of California Press.

Zola, Irving. 1966. Culture and symptoms—an analysis of patients' presenting complaints. *American Sociological Review* 31, no. 5 (October): 615–30.

# Index

adolescents: dependency of, 138–39, 167, 201n11; express distress through the body, 149, 166; liminal status as clinical actors, 12; metaphors help make complex concepts more understandable to, 43; personhood diagnostics holds salience for, 60; "stickiness" used as "soft" diagnosis for, 92–93; use of "off-label" drugs to treat chronic pain in, 69. *See also* parents

akathisia, 77–78

"all in your head" metaphor: generates response that is not generally positive, 180; interpreted to mean absence of concrete explanation for pain, 42, 52, 53; multiple meanings of, 33; neuroscience has shifted meaning of, 5, 31, 42, 108; used when diagnostic tests are inconclusive, 4; use may cause harm to patient, 182

Anspach, Renee, 111

Argawal, Nadia (pseud.), 105

Aristotle, 33

Asperger syndrome, 94, 95, 96, 101, 107, 161

Ativan, 121

attention deficit disorder (ADD), 97

attention deficit/hyperactivity disorder (ADHD), 95

Austin, John L., 180–81, 190n58

autism, 92, 96, 104, 107, 181

Azande, 6–7

Barnes, Nancy (pseud.), 89, 92

Baron-Cohen, Simon, 107

Bateson, Gregory, 138

Beard, George M., 140, 142, 168

Beecher, Henry, 15

Belkin, Shelly (pseud.), 91

Bergman, Tess (pseud.), 24–25, 26, 173

Bergmann, Harvey (pseud.), 44–47

Berlant, Lauren, 30

biomedicine: as cultural system, 7; definition of, 188n13; explanation in can reproduce class biases, 84; failure of explanation in, 14, 15; four dimensions of explanation in, 7–9; hierarchies of referral in, 18

blame: diagnosis of stickiness shifts locus of, 104; mind-body dualism and, 11, 26; neurobiology of pain alleviates patients of, 42–43, 47, 76; parents as focus of if child doesn't improve, 103, 115–16, 128, 131; personhood diagnostics do not relieve patients from, 81, 85; shifted with discourse context, 179

body: computer/machine metaphor for, 7, 49–50, 53, 195n28; distress expressed through, 149, 166; mind-body dualism,